Chi Power Plus:

Scientific Premium Company - USA

Published by Velocity Group Publishing

PO Box 9516 Hamilton, NJ 08650   www.chipower.com   www.mindforcesecrets.com

Chi Power Plus

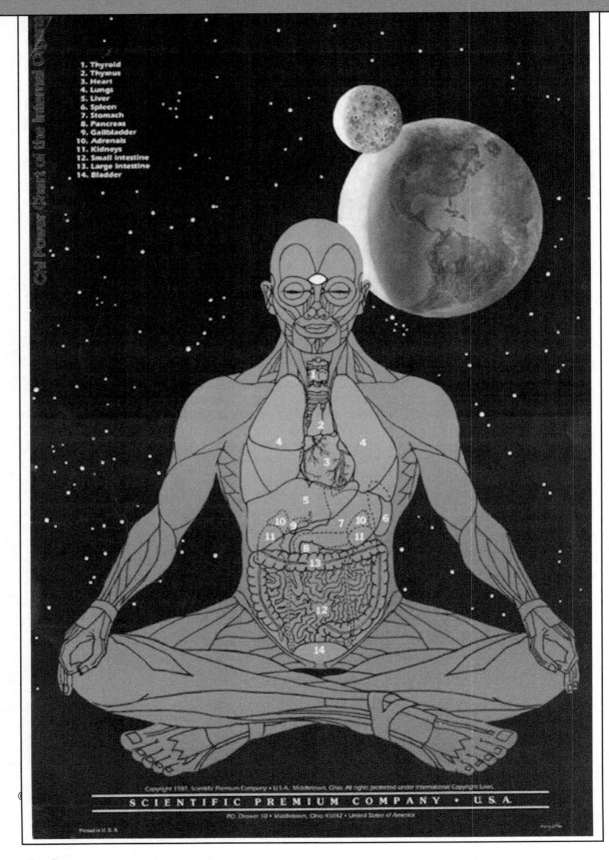

Contents

Chi Power Plus:... 1

By Scientific Premium Company - USA 1
   Published by Velocity Group Publishing 1

BREATHING WITH CHI POWER....................................... 8

YIN AND YANG.. 10

GRAVITY AND ANTIGRAVITY 10
   NEGATIVE ION FORCE 10
   POSITIVE ION FORCE 10
   THE OBJECT OF CHI POWER PRACTICE IS TO 11

Yin/Yang BALANCE 11
   YIN/YANG BALANCE AND YOUR DIET 12

CHI POWER & SPC-USA ACUPRESSURE............................... 12
   FOCUS TEST 13

ANIMAL CONTROL 14
   ATTRACT BIRDS 14
   THE MARTIAL ARTS BOW 15

LIFTING A BOWL OF WATER WITH CHI POWER 15

STRIKING WITH YANG CHI POWER............................. 15

FOCUSED YANG CHI FOR BREAK TEST 16

SELECTIVE BREAKS WITH YANG CHI 17

RINGING THE CHIMES WITH YANG CHI 18

KEEPING WARM 18

KEEPING COOL 19

VISUALIZATION OF INTERNAL ORGANS 19

USING CHI POWER FOR PROTECTION.......................... 20
   THE SPIRITUAL MESSAGE 20
   CHI POWER AWARENESS 21

ANGELS, YIN AND YANG 21
    TIME CONTROL 22

CREATED LIGHT, DARKNESS, TIME, AND SPEED.................. 22

CHI POWER IN THE DIMENSION OF TIME........................... 24
    LEVELS OF EXISTENCE..24

Audio Tape Record Your Own Voice 25
    PART 1 25
    PART II 25
       MOVE TO YOUR PRACTICE HANGING OBJECT 27
    PART III..27
    PART IV 32
    NOW DO THE STRETCHING EXERCISES 33
    FOCUS EXERCISE - MOVE STRAW.................................34
    FOCUS EXERCISE - EYE PRACTICE 35
    FOCUS EXERCISE - EXTINGUISH A CANDLE WITH YOUR EYES 36
    FOCUS EXERCISE - THROW YOUR YANG CHI TO EXTINGUISH THE FLAME 37

FOCUS EXERCISE - TIME CONTROL 38

BUILDING A CHI POWER VOICE 38

PROBLEM SOLVING.. 39

SAMPLE CHI POWER PLUS PROGRAM............................ 40

CHI POWER TIPS.. 41

"INNER CIRCLE" & "CLOSED DOOR" 54

Secret trainings and techniques that until now have never been shared with anyone other than our closest, most personal students 54

Scientific Premium Company- USA.................................. 54

Introduction.. 55
    What is the Inner Circle?..55
    What is behind the Closed Door?..................................55

Chapter 1: What is Chi? 59
    The Physics behind the Mysticism 59

Chi and the Human Body..59

Chi and the Brain..59

Electricity & Chi: One and the Same **62**

Bioelectricity...62

Bioelectricity and the Body 63

Chi and the Body Continued 64

Chi, the Inner Circle, and You!..**64**

Chapter 2: The SPC Method **65**

Mental Preparation **65**

Ascending Euphoria..65

Affirmations and Autosuggestion 65

Chi Distillation **66**

Physical Exercises **66**

Bloodwashing 66

Standing Meditation...66

Lying Down Meditation..67

Micro/Macro Cosmic Orbits [month 3]..67

Chapter 3: The Inner Circle **68**

Welcome **68**

About the IC..**68**

The Nature of Chi..**68**

Circular Chi vs. Linear Chi..68

Three Stages of Chi..69

Light Chi & Heavy Chi...70

Nutrition and Chi Power..**71**

Chapter 4: Inner Circle Curriculum **72**

Techniques and Building Blocks..**72**

Telekinesis and Psi abilities **72**

Using Chi to Bend Metal 72

Got Skills?...73

Sensing Objects...73

Sensing Colors 73

OBE 74

Remote Viewing & Astral Projection 74

Advanced Healing Techniques 75

Transferring Energy: Hot and Cold Temperatures 75

The Law of Attraction **76**
Pheromones **76**

Pheromones: "Yin and Yang" 77

Pheromones and Chi 77

Pheromones and the Inner Circle 78

Emotional Content **78**
Chi Training Partner **80**

Chapter 5: Inner Circle Community **81**
Questions & Answers Sessions and Topics **81**

Q & A Session 1 81

Q & A Session 2 83

Q & A Session 3 83

Q & A Session 4 85

Q & A Session 5 86

Q & A Session 6 88

Q & A Session 7 90

Q & A Session 8 92

Q & A Session 9 94

Interviews with Certified Instructors **96**

Sifu Michael Allen 96

Sifu Benjamin Richardson 96

Sifu Andrei Biesinger 98

Sifu Charles Dragoo 98

Sifu Don Brown 98

Chapter 6: The Closed Door **99**
Behind the Closed Door **99**
Two 6 Month Intensive Training Systems **99**

The 1st 6 Months (Form Chi)...99

Closed Door: Module One (Release of Advanced Chi DVD Volume 3).........100

Closed Door: ModuleTwo (Body Breathing)..100

Closed Door: Module Three (Advanced OBE)..100

Closed Door: Module Four (Wall to Wall Exercise)...............................100

Closed Door: Module Five (Advanced Circle Training)..........................100

Closed Door: Module Six (Levitation 101)...101

The 2nd 6 Months Closed Door System (Super Set..............................101

Training)..101

Closed Door: Module Seven (Effective Control Methods)......................101

Closed Door: Module Eight (Liquid Chi)...101

Closed Door: Module Nine (Hypnotic Devices Training)......................101

Closed Door: Module Ten (Super Set Variations)................................102

Closed Door: Module Eleven (Fractal Images)....................................102

Closed Door: Module Twelve (Integration of All Techiques)...............102

Scientific Premium Company-USA Products 103

Chi Power Plus..103

Advanced Chi Training System...103

Mind Force Collection of Esoteric Products 103

- Move objects without touching them
- Move an object with your eyes only
- Extinguish a candle flame with your eyes
- Learn how you can make select breaks
- Control animals, birds, fish, with Chi o
- Move faster than a cat with Chi Power
- Try to lift a bowl of water with Chi o
- Ring the chimes with a Chi throw

BREATHING WITH CHI POWER

Often when new practitioners begin to practice SPC'USA Chi Power, they will overlook the most vital information in the Chi Plus Book: how to breathe correctly. They will then begin to question if this is another hoax. So please, read the entire book first. Follow all of the instructions. Everything works! And it will probably work much better than you expect. We are still getting calls offeats that someone does that surprise us. After you have fully read the book, and listened to the Tape, make your own recording. You can't learn the art of focus without it! Deep-breathing, called Chi Gung, increases the energy level in the body. It adds body chemicals from your glands, as well as more fully oxygenating the blood, giving the muscles an extra measure of power. By directing the enhanced blood to the tips of your fingers, your kinetic or electrical energy (Chi, pronounced Chee) can be forcefully expelled outside your body. Note: Chi is often called Ki, Qi, Ji, Chy, or Kee, but it is all the same thing.

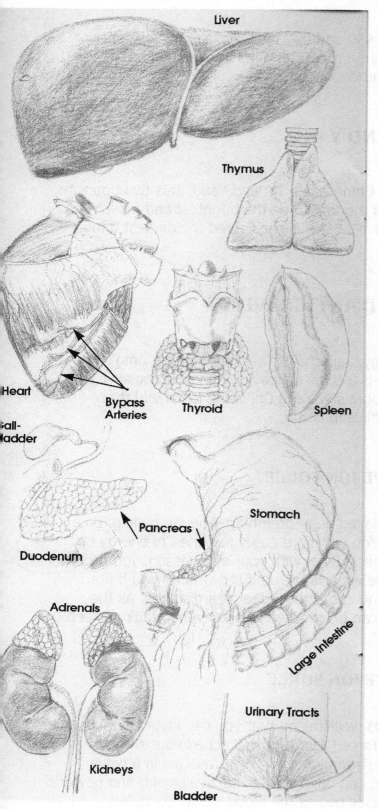

Liver

Thymus

Heart

Bypass Arteries

Thyroid

Spleen

Gall-bladder

Duodenum

Pancreas

Stomach

Adrenals

Large Intestine

Urinary Tracts

Kidneys

Bladder

Your Chi Point is located about 2" below

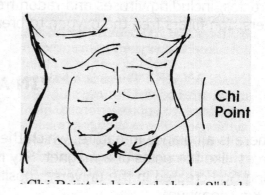

Chi Point

your navel (belly button). Draw your breath in slowly thru your nose, downward thru your lungs and intestines to your Chi Point. Your actual breath extends only to the bottom of your lungs (see #4 on Poster). But the electrical energy force (Chi) can be directed to any part of your body. The location of your Chi Point is so your Chi will pass thru the massive blood supply in your abdominal area. During relaxed breathing, your abdominal muscles should expand. Do not attempt to regulate your breath by counting. It causes great confusion to the art of learning to focus your mind thru developed reflex action. Chi Gung should be practiced at your natural breath rhythm as if you are deep-sleeping. Exhaling the waste products, which your blood has carried to your lungs, is as important as inhaling the oxygen. Chi Power practice should be performed in an oxygen-rich atmosphere with few air pollutants. If you are indoors, you should have live plants in the room (especially the sleeping room) because the plants produce oxygen. Air purifiers, such as electronic ionizers, are now available for home, office, or automobile. They emit negative ions which attach themselves to air pollutants and remove them from the air, thus freeing the oxygen molecules. They are highly recommended for use where practicing Chi

Gung. A good one can be purchased for $50 and up, and will clean microscopic particles, including viruses and radon from a room. Ion filters are NOT mere air filters. Ion filters free the oxygen to breathe.

YIN AND YANG

There is a balance in nature, which the Chinese call Yin and Yang. It is two opposite forces, like the poles of a magnet. Sky is thought to be the brightest and most Yang thing God created in the universe (positive). Earth is considered the darkest thing, or Yin (negative).

GRAVITY AND ANTIGRAVITY

Your body is powered by electrical energy, called Chi. Yin Chi (negative ions) attracts or will draw an object to you. It is a force of gravity. Yang Chi (positive ions) pushes objects away. It is a force of antigravity. Yang Chi is the ion shield that protects your body, and powers your strikes in battle.

NEGATIVE ION FORCE

This should be your usual state while relaxed deep-breathing. The ion pulling force (Yin Chi) will draw objects toward you. You will more easily feel the Chi energy of others and increase your mental awareness. Even with your eyes closed, you should feel the movement of others. This will be especially true if they intend you harm. They will be creating a Yang Chi force you can actually feel at a distance. As the Yang Chi force gets very near you, you can be shocked awake even if you're asleep.

POSITIVE ION FORCE

It is very important to have your body so well-trained that you can instantly focus to any part of your body. The positive ion force (Yang Chi) will act as your shield. Forced, vocal, deep breaths, along with strongly tensing your muscles in a wave from your toes up thru your entire body, can build your protective shield, and power your strikes in battle. Tensing your muscles begins the blood vessel shrinking process. Your glands then will release chemicals to help shrink your entire vascular system (about 60,000 miles long). The shrinking of your blood vessels greatly speeds the flow of blood cells. Electrical energy and heat are generated by the dynamic action of the blood cells as they rotate and speed in orbit throughout your body. The stars and planets create gravity this same way, as they rotate and speed in orbit thru the heavens. You can actually control one of the most powerful forces that God created, because you were created in His Image, not the image of an animal! Animals do not have your powers.

THE OBJECT OF CHI POWER PRACTICE IS TO

(1) **Build your breathing into a natural deep-breathing habit.** The number of breaths you normally take per minute should decrease.

(2) **Keep your internal organs in a constant state of balance.**

(3)**Increase the size of your blood vessels.** Your ability to greatly enlarge and shrink your blood vessels, naturally and without drugs, is the key to great Chi Power.

(4) **Increase proportionally, the volume of blood your body will hold.** This requires traditional type exercise, as well as Chi Power practice. It is the secret of endurance and great strength.

(5) **Teach you to focus your thoughts instantly to any spot on or in your body, for the purpose of tensing or relaxing your muscles.** This combination will greatly increase your mental and physical awareness. God commands us to rest, as well as to labor. By your continual affirmation to trust God, He will forewarn you of danger, expose untruths, better your life quality in every manner, and increase your lifespan. Speak out for God, and God will reward you. Test Him! That's His Written Promise!

Yin/Yang BALANCE

Yin/Yang balance is essential for good health. Yin/Yang muscle control (tensing and relaxing). Yin/Yang breathing. People inhale oxygen and exhale carbon dioxide. Plants "inhale" carbon dioxide and "exhale" oxygen. Certain foods are Yang foods, that will raise the body temperature. Yin foods will lower the body temperature. The pharmaceutical companies have exploited this knowledge, to develop chemicals which offer cures for nearly every disease. But many people now rely solely upon these chemicals and become addicted. This throws the natural healing force of the body out of balance. All medicine is simply an aid to the natural healing powers in your own body, and should be treated as such. The Spirit of God is not even considered by many physicians. But that Spirit is essential for healing and keeping healthy both body and mind. Your body is considered the temple of the Spirit. God, Who humbled Himself to become flesh, took away the corruptible spirit of mankind and replaced it with His Holy Spirit, remaking us into Image Beings, so that we may have power to resist temptation of those things that are hurtful to the flesh. This Holy Spirit is known as the Comforter to those who believe in the Savior. There will always be a way to escape temptation! To please God, giving part of one's time for exercise in order to properly care for this fleshly temple is essential. Moderation in exercise, eating, drinking, and work, is required. Both the quality and quantity of food should be carefully considered, in order for the temple to be useful. It is not the same for everyone. The air that you breathe should be reasonably free of pollutants and filled with oxygen. In a city atmosphere, oxygen can be added with live leafy plants in your practice area.

YIN/YANG BALANCE AND YOUR DIET

Your ancestors helped form your body by what they ate and drank. You have the obligation to eat foods that are nutritionally balanced. Scriptures forbid the eating of fat or blood. Your body will often develop allergies to foods for your own protection. You should choose foods, even though they may be higher priced, that are fresh and good in all aspects. Better to go a bit hungry than to suffer the many viruses caused by spoiled food. Be sure to thoroughly wash meat, poultry, fish, fresh fruits and vegetables, just before eating them, to remove harmful germs or chemicals.

CHI POWER & SPC-USA ACUPRESSURE

The injured person should Chi Gung breathe to ease the pain. Before using acupressure, first rub your hands together for friction warmth. Then place them in the chest level praying position and draw Chi heat into your hands. The heat from your hands can penetrate deeper to quickly relax the constricted muscles. The muscle constriction causes pain by constricting the blood flow into the injured area, thus causing a muscular spasm in that area. The result of the muscle spasm is pain that ranges in intensity from mild to severe. Simple pressure over knotted muscles and muscle-stretching exercises will then remove the pain permanently. Ice slows the flow of blood and will prolong pain.

Currently in China, it is reported a Chi Power practitioner is using Chi Power with Acupressure to cause paralysis to disappear. He has had much success. The patients are those whom the Medical Doctors have declared hopeless! Anyone can develop

Chi Power. If you are infirm (physically unable to stand on your feet), lie flat on your back, and follow the directions. Mentally direct all your strength to that end. Also get help from someone who will use Acupressure. It is easier to develop Chi Power with an empty stomach and pure concentrated thought. Chi Practice is best performed after a night's sleep, and before eating (food digestion requires a large amount of your blood).

If you have trouble sleeping, practice the Chi before retiring for the night. This is an individual or private family practice, so the voice of most authority should should not be used in a school atmosphere. The sharp command discipline of an instructor may prevent communication with your Creator. You need to record the directions on an audio cassette, or have someone else read them to you while you go thru it; so that you can more fully concentrate on what you are doing. Your powers of concentration and focus will build with regular practice.

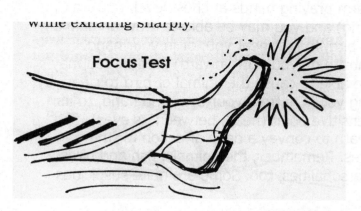

FOCUS TEST

(1) **Breathe Chi Gung rhythmically.**
(2) **Direct your thoughts to a portion of your body. You choose the part.**
(3) **Feel that body part with your senses.**
(4) **Tense it. Imagine that part to be as hard as stone. Then with a quick twist, you are able to direct your Chi outward from that spot, while exhaling sharply.**

We have deliberately left the body part for the user's discretion. Examples:

(A) In order to kick with more force and provide maximum protection for your foot, you would direct the Chi with concentrated thought to a small part of your kicking foot.

(B) If in danger of receiving an injury to your leg, you would flex the muscle while slightly twisting and direct the Chi to the specific part being attacked, to minimize the damage.

(C) When throwing a punch: You would direct the Chi to the open palm. Then slightly twist your hand with fingers tightly together to build Chi and to harden your hand for your own protection. (See your Martial Arts instructor for specific directions of how to protect your fingers when using an open hand punch.)

ANIMAL CONTROL

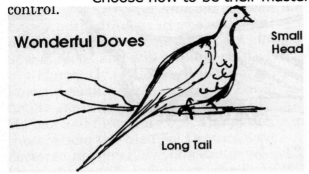

Wonderful Doves

Small Head

Long Tail

control.

Creatures understand your thoughts and intent. You are their master or their foe. Choose now to be their master. Don't abuse them, but cultivate them. Build your Yin Chi (warm praying hands at chest level, relaxed Chi Breathing) and you may be able to draw an animal, fish, or bird, to rest near you, or in your hand. Concentrate on your Yin (inward) breath. You may even be able to cause the animal or bird to sleep, by directing your Chi from your eyes and hand, to its heat-sensitive point (head, between its eyes). You must learn to convey a deep affection for the creatures. Remember, the animals, fish and birds have personalities, too. Some are quite suspicious and hard to control.

ATTRACT BIRDS

Doves are not the same as pigeons. About the size of a pigeon, they have a small head, a long tail, and make a distinctive cooing sound. They always foretell good times. Don't use Yang Chi on these wonderful birds. They help the farmer by eating weed seed. They do not eat farm grain. Use Yin Chi to draw them, and other birds you want, to your area.

REPEL DIRTY BIRDS, such as starlings, greckles, pigeons, or other pest-type birds, by placing your hands together in the praying position at chest level. Direct your Chi to your hands until your hands are warm. Tighten your gut, then push hands together hard, while focusing your eyes on the bird. Then sharply exhale your breath. This same Yang Chi technique should work on animals of any size, and cause them to move away if stationary, or alter their course away from you. Larger animals may require the use of your Chi Voice and the *Joshua Jericho Shout 'YAH-HWAH" (on Tape) while throwing your Chi to repel them. Remember, you must learn to build strong Chi Power first, or it may not be effective.   *Joshua 6:20 in the Bible

THE MARTIAL ARTS BOW

The chest level praying position, with eyes directed at other people, can now have a much different intention! Give respect to those who deserve respect. Really bow only to God. Keep your eyes open when facing other people. Even teachers. You must learn to trust only God. Even the best teachers are human. But, everyone can teach you something. We were all created in the Image of God. But none of us are yet...Gods!

LIFTING A BOWL OF WATER WITH CHI POWER

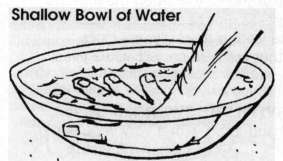
Shallow Bowl of Water

Use a shallow bowl and partly fill it with water. After building your Chi, place your hand under the water in the bowl. With each of your fingers extended, touch the lower sides of the bowl. Your fingertips can press against the sides of the bowl with enough pressure so that you can then lift the bowl. Begin with a lightweight bowl that won't break if dropped. Be prepared to clean up water spills. This is a very difficult test. Only the strongest Chi Power practitioners can perform it.

STRIKING WITH YANG CHI POWER

Do this only when you have learned the art of focus thru much practice using the SPC-USA Chi Power Chart. Your mind must learn to focus automatically to each muscle. Repetition) along with the deep-breathing, is very necessary to learn the art of focus. Without regular practice, your body will not respond in a predictable manner; and should you attempt these break tests, serious personal injury could be the result. We strongly advise against the break tests until you have complete confidence in your mental focus abilities. When you strike with Yang Chi Power, you take with the strike electrical energy, that gives more power to your strikes. This power is able to penetrate deep within the object of your strike. Since Chi is smaller than an atom, it can penetrate even concrete blocks, bricks, or wooden boards, even thru your eyeglasses (if you wear them).

FOCUSED YANG CHI FOR BREAK TEST

Use a wooden sword to break a one-inch thick board. (1) Prop each end of a board on a block. Focus your eyes on the center of the board. (2) Build your Chi. (3) Inhale to your Chi Point and hold. (4) Exhale sharply, as you direct your Chi to the point of impact against your sword. The board should break. The sword should stop exactly thru the thickness of the object of strike. Not a fraction more nor less!

We do not recommend toughening hands, except by finger pushup exercise. Your Chi should be sufficient to protect you. We believe you can keep your hands very sensitive, to feel others' Chi or even flowing air. Destruction of your surface blood vessels and nerve system can cause arthritic crippling to your hands. You would not think of toughening your elbow or forehead,
would you? If you choose to break with your hands, be very sure of your focused Chi Power first. That is why we recommend a wooden sword as a first practice instrument. We recommend that you practice finger pushups, to harden the muscles of your hands. Then wear leather gloves for hand breaks. For head breaks, wear a cloth or leather headband. The Chi will pass thru the leather as easily as it does eyeglasses, boards, or concrete blocks, and the leather will help protect you against splinters.

ONLY AFTER YOU HAVE ACHIEVED SUCCESS WITH THE SWORD, begin to break with your hands. Use the gloved fist of your hand. Start with a very wide one-inch thick pine board. Cut a short wide strip from the board. The pine board grain (lines of growth) should be placed so that when you strike, you will strike with the grain parallel to your strike. If you strike against the grain, you may suffer ...iem). injury. Exhale sharply as you strike.

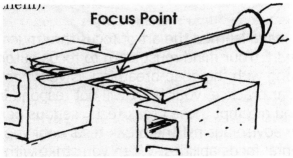

Focus Point

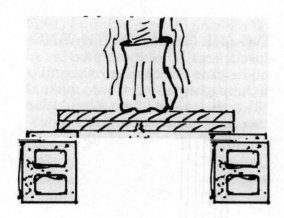

SELECTIVE BREAKS WITH YANG CHI

Use two boards. Try to break the bottom board, but not the top. Your strike should stop exactly at the bottom depth of your top board. Your Chi will then continue to the exact depth of the selected board and cause it to break. This takes concentration and practice. Add boards and focus your Chi to break a specific board from a stacked pile, by stopping your Yang Chi at that selected level.

Yang Chi Fist Strike

You may wish to graduate to shallow cement slabs or bricks. Try putting stress oi the object you wish to selectively break with a pro-strike. This is a dangerous practice, even for highly trained Chi Power practitioners; but well worth learning, because you learn to exactly control your Chi Power. Again, use a glove to protect your very valuable hands.

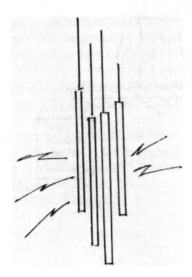

RINGING THE CHIMES WITH YANG CHI

Purchase or build a set of very lightweight wind chimes. As you regularly pass by them, throw your Chi to make them chime. The visual and audio stimulation can cause you much pleasure and joy!

KEEPING WARM

While Chi Gung breathing, direct the Chi thru your nose and down your spine, which contains major nerves. A heat build up should occur and you can actually feel the heat as it passes down your spine. Then breathe outwardly up from your Chi Point slowly thru pursed lips. Blood-vessel-shrinking chemicals can be drawn from any and all of your glands, from the pituitary near your brain to gonad glands for giving life.

KEEPING COOL

In this case, by cool, we mean keeping your temper. Forcefully direct your Yang Chi breath from your Chi point out the top of your head. The Chi will excite the pituitary gland located at the back center of your skull. This works also to calm your anxieties, or lessen your grief. This technique can also help you to sleep. Another technique is to hold the top of your ear between your forefinger and thumb for a few moments. This will usually cause a yawn. Asthma patients can stop the muscle spasm that prevents normal breathing by pushing the skin with a finger over and under the collarbone joint (sternum) at the base of the neck.

VISUALIZATION OF INTERNAL ORGANS

The purpose of the Chi Power Poster and the detailed drawings is to help you visualize the location and shape of your internal organs, in order for you to direct your Chi to that location. The visualization methods described are for the purpose of restoring the natural chemical action within your internal organs.

First, examine carefully each internal organ shown and numbered on the poster, and its relative position. Where shown on the body drawing, the broken lines indicate those organs or parts of organs located behind other organs. Your spleen is located under your left front ribcage. Your pancreas begins near the liver, extends behind your stomach and in front of your kidneys. Your gallbladder is behind your liver, extending above and to the right of your pancreas. Beginning under your back ribs, your adrenal glands are located on top of each kidney. Your kidneys are on each side of your backbone.

The thymus, once thought to be of little use, is important in building additional energy, as well as keeping your immune system functioning properly. Your liver and spleen perform similar functions to filter your blood. You're probably already familiar with the functions of the other organs.

Then, study the drawings of the positions of the hands that appear within the recording instructions. This Chi Power exercise should be performed while sitting, preferably in the cross-legged position, with back straight for easy breathing. Place your hand over each organ as the name is mentioned. Force the Chi into each organ, to open the blood flow to the organ. By the forced deep-breathing, you also force oxygen into the blood vessels that feed your internal organs. Then direct the Chi flow out thru each organ.

Version 2.0

USING CHI POWER FOR PROTECTION

Simply by breathing Chi Gung and progressively tensing the muscles of your body, you can increase and direct the blood and Chi flow to any part of your body that you choose. Muscular flex (contraction), along with the pumping movement of legs and arms, will increase the Chi and bloodflow. The rest of your body can be relaxed, while you progressively flex your muscles in a particular part. Look at the inside of your left wrist. By flexing your left forearm and hand, making a fist and opening it, and pumping your arm, you can increase the size of the blood vessels in your left wrist to be visibly larger than the vessels of your right wrist which is still at rest. Using this type of Chi Gung breathing, flexing, and pumping action, you can direct Chi Power to any part of your body: your hand, foot, elbow, etc. You control the thought as well as the power. Direct it where you will, but use caution.

Your Chi Power can be far more forceful than you may imagine. You are able to flex your muscles to become as hard as stone. This requires mentally directed thought to a degree that is self-hypnotic. But unlike hypnosis that is directed by another, YOU control the thought. Everyone is in a hypnotic state, while being fully conscious, as they ride a bicycle or even watch television. The hypnotic thoughts will affect you. Choose very carefully what you see or hear. Repeating meaningless phrases or sounds (such as mantras) can do you harm by wasting valuable focus practice.

Your mind, like unexercised muscles, will lose strength. An unexercised mind loses its flexibility of thought. It can continually return to an unhealthy thought to destroy your mind and body. A visitor to a mental hospital spoke to the administrator on the way out. The visitor said, "All the patients seemed very normal to me. Many of them were highly intelligent." "Yes", said the administrator, "they may seem normal, but all of their conversation is about themselves. That is what brought them here. They could only think of themselves." Looking inward leads to self-pity and insanity.

THE SPIRITUAL MESSAGE

It Is the most important to strengthen your mind as well as your internal organs. This Chi Practice is to establish and keep a right relationship with your Creator. With practice, you also learn the art of focus. You should be able to focus your mind instantly where you wish. Along with the focus of your mind goes the living energy called Chi. Learn to direct the Chi to any object as an extension of your arms or eyes. You will be amazed at your new accuracy. God then directs your aim.

CHI POWER AWARENESS

Chi can help you improve your awareness of what may be impending danger. Begin practicing awareness: Close your eyes, close one hand into a fist and hold out your other open hand. Move it slowly back and forth to see if you can feel (without touching them) solid objects that are a few inches, then a few feet distant from you. Concentrate. You should feel a temperature change in the tips of your fingers. If you do not feel a change, build your Chi Power and try it again.

Practice Relaxed Chi Breathing continually and you will also feel the presences of other people and their movements. Try it: Sit relaxed with your back to another. As the person moves, you will feel a temperature change on your head, ears, or back of your neck. With Chi Power awareness, there are no surprise attacks! Even if you sleep and a hostile intruder bumps your Chi, you will suddenly waken. Remember to think of the Chi Relaxation, as well as the Chi Buildup, for self-defense. When you become adept at both, you will often find it easier to relax a muscle away from impending danger than to tense it against it.

With regular SPC USASA Chi Power practice, your mind can develop enough focus of muscular constriction that you can cause a wave of constriction to flow from your toes to the tips of your fingers in an instant. The potential power that can be generated in this manner is truly awesome! Be extremely careful, and learn to control your temper. Speak softly because your voice is also filled with Chi Power. This Chi Power from your voice can cause illness. People have been reported to knock a bird from the air with voice!

ANGELS, YIN AND YANG

The ion shield is only partly protecting you. Even though light is considered Yang, the light causes a Yin Chi attraction. A Yin Angel of Light can shield you from injury. But Yang Angels of Deception try to trick you. They conduct "sting" operations to cause you to do hurtful things to yourself and others. God permits this because we are given freewill choices. But there is always a terrible price to pay, so that you will correct your behavior. The Yang Angels are often called demons. They are in spirit form.

Often, the spirits will have invaded the body of a human being. An example is found in the New Testament account of Jesus casting out demons from the man called Legion. Satan was a serpent. He wanted to be like an Image Being, such as we are, but God said NO! Satan still pretends he is a man or woman, because he is able to invade the thoughts of people. But God said that we humans are His Image Beings, and we are to become Partners with God.

Yin Angels of Protection are led by God's Holy Spirit to warn you of Yang deception and danger. The Yin Angels are able to choose both the time and the place for "accidents" to happen to you. The accidents are not by chance. This is the way God renders justice on Earth. God is much more merciful than men or women, so heed those feelings that warn you. But use reasoned thought to make decisions, not simply your feelings. Examine the thought message very carefully to see if it is from Yin or Yang. Let your conscience help guide you. Faith is trusting God and not yourself. You can be an easy target for Yang deception if you trust in just your own abilities. With God, all things are possible. God wishes you good continually. To know God is to love Him.

TIME CONTROL

While in the Chi Power state of generating a positive ion force, you will see things moving in slow motion. The strength of the Yang Chi force that you create will slow the movement of time for you. Often in a near death experience, you will see an actual time reversal. Many people report seeing their entire life flash before their eyes.

This gives the Chi Practitioner a very great advantage. To others, you will seem to move with blinding speed. The late scientist Albert Einstein, in his Speed of Light Theory, stated that time stops when a moving mass reaches the speed of light. Light speed is also a force of gravity (Yang Chi). Other scientists proved the time theory is true by using a jet airplane and two atomic clocks. Time on the speeding jet greatly slowed, in comparison to the stationary clock on Earth. A person who practices Chi Power sees this scientific principle in practical application.

CREATED LIGHT, DARKNESS, TIME, AND SPEED

The speed of light is thought to be about 186,000 miles per second. But this is a flawed theory. (That is the speed of some reflected light, measured from the Moon.) When an atomic molecule leaves a burning mass, such as the Sun, it is in a high state of agitation (see drawing below).

Then as the molecule loses heat, its state of agitation slows; and the light that was caused by the agitated molecule begins to dim. It also begins to slow in speed. So the speed of light is a variable speed. The molecule will eventually cool and float as a gas molecule in space, and will be affected by gravitational forces.

Path of Element Molecule (Light)

As an example, though extremely lightweight, the molecule of light can be diverted to a very erratic path by forces of gravity from celestial bodies as it travels thru space. The cold molecules will fuse to form a 'wall" at the edge of a star's gravitational field. The wall is held in place just as the Earth is held in place by the mutual pull of gravity between the Sun and the Earth.

A cold fusion of molecular gas is formed like water in a cloud of gas. With the fusion, heat is created. The heat causes movement of other free-floating molecular bodies which in turn cool to form even more complex molecules (minerals) to form mass. This mass forms a layered wall at the edge of the celestial equator of a star system. A similar wall is formed around the planets in our Solar System, as well as our Milky Way Galaxy.

The most famous of these walls are the rings around the Planet Saturn and around the "Sombrero Galaxy". Because of its huge size, the wall around a star system or a galaxy is called a "Ring World". A molecular mass of any size acts the same way. All create both a Yin and a Yang force of gravity. The smallest mineral is hydrogen. When hydrogen fuses with another hydrogen molecule it becomes helium. As the molecule becomes more complex thru fusion, it takes on new character.

Iron is 26 molecules of hydrogen fused together. Uranium has 92 molecules of hydrogen fused together. Uranium is very unstable (comes apart easily). Uranium is used in fission (separation of molecular or atomic mass) that also creates heat. Our current atomic power electric generators are creating energy by a fission reaction. The fission creates radio activity that can harm or help people, depending upon its use. In a bomb it is destructive. But in small amounts it can help the growth of plant life, or kill cancerous cells within a living body.

Our future atomic power electric generators will be fusion generators. The only known byproducts effusion are heat and minerals. These minerals will usually be water or gas. Some of the gas formed could be quite poisonous. Unless carefully controlled, any type of energy created by Yin and Yang gravity forces has the potential for harm. This includes your personal use of it!

The so-called "Light Year of Time" is as fictional as the speed of light. However, the forces of gravity can increase or slow time to give the illusion of speed. "Time" and "speed" are both illusions of the mind used by God to create levels of existence. God sees light, darkness, and time, as created forces to be controlled and used for heavenly purposes. (SPC -USA's Prolepsis History of Chi Power booklet explains more about created anti-light (darkness), and anti-sound. Contact us at www.chipower.com if you have not already read this thought provoking manuscript.

CHI POWER IN THE DIMENSION OF TIME

Other planets and other star systems are for human expansion. And, they are so numerous they are beyond our ability to count. There are billions of stars injust our own small Milky Way Galaxy. And the number of galaxies are beyond counting. The astronomers are astounded by the order within the universe, and the spacing between galaxies.

LEVELS OF EXISTENCE

Fall within the dimension called time. They can and do overlap each other. Prophets, often called Seers, can and do see events in historic perspective. The Christian Book of Revelations was seen as a vision by John, the Apostle of Christ. John saw the entire history of Earth, from its first creation by God, thru the birth of God from the Holy Spirit's conception into a woman, to Earth's final conclusion as the completed Garden. Because many religions can't believe God could or would become flesh and sacrifice Himself for the forgiveness of sin for anyone who believes in His Grace, there is still much division in the world. Many wars have been fought to retain political power within a religious group.

Nationalities and races must merge. This is why God directs sons and daughters to leave their parents. There are many good reasons why incest or family intermarrying are illegal. God wishes for the world to be repopulated with people who are not Atheists, but believers in One God. The completion of the Earth Garden must be done by people who have mastered the powers that God gave to every human, but not to animals. God is very patient. He will give Atheists all the time they need to determine His existence. Some of it will not be very pleasant. It has been said, there are few Atheists in foxholes!

Audio Tape Record Your Own Voice

<u>WHEN YOU HAVE READ THE ENTIRE BOOK, AND LISTENED TO THE TAPE, YOU ARE READY TO MAKE YOUR RECORDING</u>.

You need to see a clock with a second hand or a stopwatch while recording, so that you leave the actual number of seconds on the tape. In PART I, use a light weight, big enough to see rise and fall. (Later on, as your strength increases, add more weight and length of time. Your Chi Power will also increase.) In PART II, your practice hanging object can be simple wind chimes or an elaborate work of mobile art. You should be far enough away that the object is moved by Chi Power and not wind. Speak every word of the instructions, except the words that are in parentheses, into the recorder. After you have your recording made, you'll play it back while you do what you say. **AUDIO TAPE RECORD YOUR OWN VOICE (BEGIN SPEAKING INTO THE RECORDER):**

PART I. First, lie on the floor on your back. Place a weight on your abdominal muscles, gut or tummy. When you breathe in, your abdomen should rise. When you breathe out, your abdomen should fall. Your breath rate should be as if deep-sleeping.

(ADD 3 MINUTES TO TAPE)...30 seconds...1 minute...I minute,30 seconds... 2 minutes...2 minutes,30 seconds...3 minutes.

PART II. Now, stand with your hands to your side in rest. Feet should be shoulder-width apart. Take a slow, deep breath. Direct your thoughts to your Chi Point, located about 2 inches below your navel. Forcefully breathe inward to your CM Point. Then force your breath out slowly thru pursed lips. Try to form a deep vocal sound as you inhale and exhale. Repeat the slow, deep breaths, feeling the Chi Point continually. Develop a comfortable, slow, deep, breath rhythm, to and from the Chi Point. Your abdomen should expand with each inhalation. You will be reminded about the breathing, so you can concentrate on fully tensing each set of muscles, to build your Chi. Begin with the big toe on your left foot. Direct your thoughts to that toe. Mentally feel its bottom; then top. Then contract it, by grabbing the floor with it. Breathe Chi Rhythm.

Now direct your thoughts to your right big toe. Feel its bottom; then top. Contract it the same way. Breathe Chi Rhythm. Now focus your attention back to the toes of your left foot. Place them in a state of tension, by strongly contracting them. Grasp the floor, and even deeper, with them. Hold the tension. Breathe Chi Rhythm. Now tense the toes of your right foot the same way. Hold the tension. Breathe Chi Rhythm.

Now tense the arch of your left foot. Hold. Tense your right arch. Hold. Breathe Chi Rhythm. Tense your left heel. Plant it deep into the floor. Hold. Tense your right heel. Hold. Breathe Chi Rhythm. Left ankle, tense. Hold. Right ankle, tense. Hold. Left calf, tense. Hold. Right calf, tense. Hold. Breathe Chi Rhythm. Left knee, tense. Hold. Right knee, tense. Hold. Breathe Chi Rhythm.

Left thigh, tense. Hold. Right thigh, tense. Hold. Buttocks, tense. Hold. Breathe Chi Rhythm. Lower back, tense. Hold. Abdominal muscles, tense. Hold. Upper back, tense. Hold. Chest, tense. Hold. Breathe Chi Rhythm.

Neck, tense. Hold. Left shoulder, tense. Hold. Right shoulder, tense. Hold. Left upper arm, tense. Hold. Right upper arm, tense. Hold. Breathe Chi Rhythm. Left elbow, tense. Hold. Right elbow, tense. Hold. Left forearm, tense. Hold. Right forearm, tense. Hold. Breathe Chi Rhythm. Left wrist, tense. Hold. Right wrist, tense. Hold. Left fingers, tense. Hold. Right fingers, tense. Hold. Left thumb, tense. Hold. Right thumb, tense. Hold. Breathe Chi Rhythm. Your entire body should now be in a state of tension. Hold that tension! Continue to breathe Chi Rhythm.

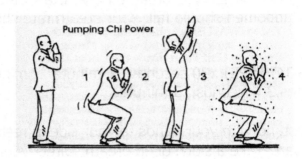

Pumping Chi Power

NOW PLACE YOUR HANDS FIRMLY TOGETHER AT EYE LEVEL, fingers tightly together, pointing upward as in praying. Exert pressure, one hand against the other. Continue the pressure as you bend your knees in a half-kneebend, feet flat on floor. At the same time, lower your hands, still pressed together, to your chest while breathing inward. Having filled your lungs, begin to expel the air thru pursed lips, making a louder sound. Do this as you begin to straighten your legs and lift your still pressed together hands to the heavens. When your praying hands are fully extended above your head and your legs are straight, you should have expelled all the air in your lungs. Then as you slowly breathe inward, lower your hands and knees again to the previous position to fill your lungs. Repeat this pumping action to build Chi.

Version 2.0

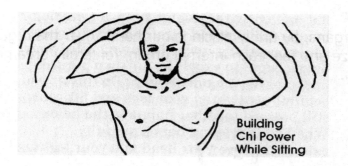

Building
Chi Power
While Sitting

MOVE TO YOUR PRACTICE HANGING OBJECT

Push-throw your Chi at the object thru your right hand, fingers cupped tightly together and thumb folded toward your palm. Direct the Chi out from the butt of your palm while using the YAH-HWAH Shout. Remember to use the circular movements for building strong throwing Chi. Then throw the Chi at the object thru your right elbow and continue to shout with each throw. Repeat with your left fingers, and left elbow. Then kick at the object with your right knee, then kick with your right foot. Now kick with your left knee; and left foot. Repeat the exercises and shouts with your fingers fully extended as a knife. Alternate and repeat several times. The object of this Practice is to throw additional bloodflow thru your joints. It also keeps you ready to defend yourself when necessary.

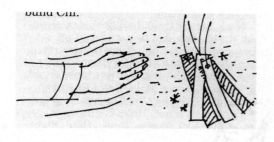

PART III

Now look at the Chi Power Poster for the locations of the organs (ADD TIME IF NECESSARY). Sit cross-legged on the floor. Now draw the Chi to your hands in praying position. Remember your inhaling should cause your tightened gut to extend slightly against the tension. To help you remember, make a deep noise when inhaling and exhaling. Direct your Chi flow, along with the statements, into and out

27

thru your internal organs, by firmly placing your hands over the organs. Close your eyes. As you visualize and feel each internal organ, forcefully breathe Chi into and out thru each organ.

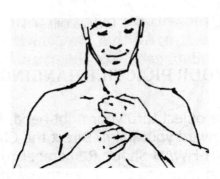

(1) Place one hand over your thyroids. Place your thumb on one side, and fingers on the other. Place your other hand over your thymus. Breathe Chi flow out thru thyroids. **THYROIDS:** My spirit is at peace, as I direct Chi Power to my internal organs...My spirit is at peace, as I direct Chi Power to my internal organs...My spirit is at peace, as I direct Chi Power to my internal organs.

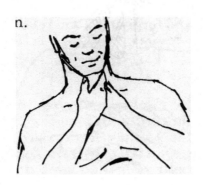

n.

(2) Place one hand over your thymus, the other just below it over your heart. Breathe Chi flow out thru thymus.

THYMUS: I am strong and courageous ...I am strong and courageous...I am strong and courageous. Now tap on the sternum, over the thymus, like Tarzan beating his chest. Tap three times with each fist. This helps to strengthen the immune system and enlarge the thymus. (3) Keep your hands in same position. Breathe Chi flow out thru heart.

HEART: I forget the bad. I remember the good. I am generous and forgiving. I am relaxed...I forget the bad. I remember the good. I am generous and forgiving. I am relaxed...I forget the bad. I remember the good. I am generous and forgiving. I am relaxed.

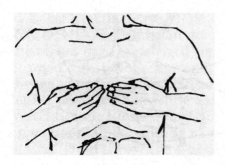

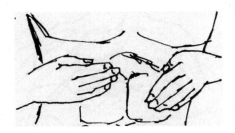

(4) Lower your hands to both sides of your ribs. Breathe Chi flow out thru lungs. **LUNGS**: I am reverent, and without fear. God is the giver of life and death. All that happens is meant for my ultimate good. For this, I am thankful...I am reverent, and without fear. God is the giver of life and death. All that happens is meant for my ultimate good. For this, I am thankful...1 am reverent, and without fear. God is the giver of life and death. All that happens is meant for my ultimate good. For this, I am thankful.

(5) Lower your hands; right hand over your liver, left hand over your spleen. Breathe Chi flow out thru liver. **LIVER:** I am happy. I am cheerful. I am kind. ..I am happy. I am cheerful. I am kind. ..I am happy. I am cheerful. I am kind.

(6) Keep hands in same position. Breathe Chi flow out thru spleen. **SPLEEN:** I am filled with faith and confidence. I expect only good. ..I am filled with faith and confidence. I expect only good...I am filled with faith and confidence. I expect only good.

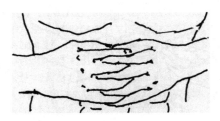

(7) Now move hands closer to each other, fingers should interface and touch, just below your ribs. Breathe Chi flow out thru stomach. **STOMACH:** I am patient and content.. .1 am patient and content...I am patient and content.

(8) Keep hands in same position. Breathe Chi flow out thru pancreas. **PANCREAS:** I look for the best in myself and others...I look for the best in myself and others...1 look for the best in myself and others.

(9) Keep hands in same position. Breathe Chi flow out thru gallbladder.
GALLBLADDER: I reach out with love and peace ...I reach out with love and peace ...I reach out with love and peace.

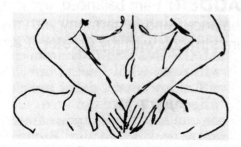

(10) Move both hands to your back, with the heels of your palms just touching your back ribcage, and fingers pointing downward on each side of your spine. Breathe Chi flow out thru adrenals. **ADRENAL GLANDS**: I am trustworthy and loyal. I am trustworthy and loyal. I am trustworthy and loyal.

(11) Keep hands in same position. Breathe Chi flow out thru kidneys. **KIDNEYS:** My internal energies are balanced .My internal energies are balanced. My internal energies are balanced.

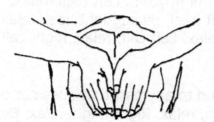

(12) Now move your hands to front of body, over small intestine. Fingers should be pointing down, with sides of hands touching each other. Breathe Chi flow out thru small intestine. **SMALL INTESTINE**: I am joyful, and filled with strength .. .I am joyful, and filled with strength .. .I am joyful, and filled with strength.

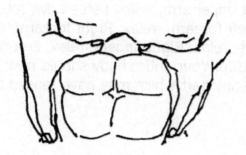

(13) Move your hands to cover your large intestine on the sides of your abdomen. Breathe Chi flow out thru large intestine. **LARGE INTESTINE:** I am clean and good. I will enjoy what I doL . .I am clean and good. I will enjoy what I doL . .I am clean and good. I will enjoy what I do!

(14) Place one hand under your crotch, the other hand over your bladder. Breathe Chi flow out thru bladder. **BLADDER:** I am balanced and in harmony with my Creator. I am happy!. . .I am balanced and in harmony with my Creator. I am happy!. . .I am balanced and in harmony with my Creator. I am happy!

PART IV

NOW GENTLY BEGIN TO RELAX YOUR BODY. Breathe as if deep sleeping. Sit with hands at rest in your lap, one hand upon the other, palms up. Be sure to keep your spine straight so that breathing is easy. Gut should extend with each inhaling breath. Again, concentrate your thoughts. Mentally visualize each muscle as you relax it. Breathe to your Chi Point in a slow, relaxed Chi Rhythm. Do not force your breath. Breathe to continually feel your Chi Point, rhythmically, as if sleeping. You now know how each muscle feels when tense. Now you are going to teach it the opposite. Each muscle will now learn to relax.

Now, relax the big toe of your left foot. Speak to it, if necessary. Relax the big toe of your right foot. Breathe Chi Rhythm. Left toes, relax. Right toes, relax. Left arch, relax. Right arch, relax. Left heel, relax. Right heel, relax. Breathe Chi Rhythm. Left ankle, relax. Right ankle, relax. Left calf, relax. Right calf, relax. Breathe Chi Rhythm.

Remember to speak out loud to any part that does not cooperate. Left knee, relax. Right knee, relax. Left thigh, relax. Right thigh, relax. Breathe Chi Rhythm. Buttocks, relax. Lower back, relax. Abdominal muscles, relax. Breathe Chi Rhythm. Upper back, relax. Chest, relax. Breathe Chi Rhythm, and speak to any part that does not stay relaxed.

Neck, relax. Left shoulder, relax. Right shoulder, relax. Breathe Chi Rhythm. Left upper arm, relax. Right upper arm, relax. Left elbow, relax. Right elbow, relax. Breathe Chi Rhythm. Left forearm, relax. Right forearm, relax. Left wrist, relax. Right wrist, relax. Left fingers, relax. Right fingers, relax. Left thumb, relax. Right thumb, relax. Breathe Chi Rhythm. Your entire body should now be completely relaxed. Remember to speak to any part which may have tensed again.

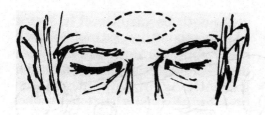

Now, look to the spot on your forehead just above your nose, the "third eye". You should see light. The light will vary in color depending upon your physical and mental condition. If you are truly relaxed and at peace, the light should be white or golden in color.

The light may now form into a shape or shapes. Some people see "visions" thru the "third eye". Don't force the vision. Allow it to open naturally. Take your time. God may show you things meant for your understanding. You may not fully comprehend the things you will see, but be patient. As time passes, God will reveal the meaning of your vision. (ADD SILENCE)...30 seconds.

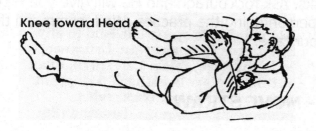

Knee toward Head

NOW DO THE STRETCHING EXERCISES

Gently begin to stretch. First, lift your chin high, to stretch your neck. Hold. Next, slowly push your chin down as far as you can toward your chest. Now very slowly roll your head to the left; then as far back as it will go; then very slowly to the right; and down toward your chest. Then reverse the process. (ADD 15 SECONDS). Next, lay on your back. Stretch your toes forward and backward as far as they will go. Relax and repeat three times. (ADD 15 SECONDS). Now, bend your left leg at the knee. With both hands, pull your knee toward your head. Try to touch your knee with your nose by moving your head to also meet your knee. Don't be discouraged if your nose does not meet your knee. The movement is only meant to stretch your muscles. Repeat the stretch with your right leg. Stretch 3 times, each leg. (ADD TIME IF NECESSARY).

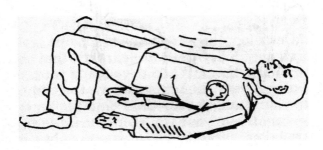

Then, with your knees bent, lift your buttocks as high as you can, and tighten your rectal orifice. Hold for 30 seconds. (ADD 30 SECONDS)...15 seconds..-30 seconds. Now stand on your feet. To improve your balance, stand on your left foot, while holding your right foot next to your groin. Try it. You can do it! (ADD 30 SECONDS)...15 seconds...30 seconds. Repeat, standing on your right foot, and holding your left foot to your groin. (ADD 30 SECONDS)...15 seconds...30 seconds. Devise your own balance exercises and length of time in training; but don't "test" God by taking foolish risks. Ask for courage and He will give you His! (You will need a focus devise for each person doing the practice. We recommend that you add all the focus exercises to your tape.)

FOCUS EXERCISE - MOVE STRAW

A soft drink straw suspended with a thread makes an excellent Chi Focus exercise device. Simply tie one end of a long thread around the middle of the straw to a level balance. Use a thumbtack, or tape, to attach the other end of the thread to the bottom side of a surface that permits the straw to freely float in the air, without friction, at your eye level.

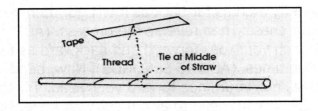

Occasionally, you will need to wipe straws with a dry cloth to clear ions that may pollute them. When developing your Chi, direct your thoughts to draw the Chi from your hand to your Chi Point.

Slowly deep-breathe to your Chi Point, and allow your abdominal muscles to expand only slightly. Do not hold your breath while concentrating. You must continue to breathe deeply and slowly (Chi Gung). With your hand about 12 inches away from the straw, and arm outstretched, gently tense your hand and arm muscles. Direct your thoughts to draw the Chi from your hand to your Chi Point. Emphasize your inward breath.

Gently beckon one end of the straw with your forefinger. The end of the straw should move toward you. You are using Yin Chi. Be sure you do not inhale or exhale directly at the straw, and that it is not being moved by any air currents in the room. You must move the straw with your Yin Chi Power only. This requires mental concentration. Now strongly tense your forefinger, and point it at one end of the straw. Push the straw with your Yang Chi, by mentally reversing your Chi flow. This takes a small mental effort. And watch the payoff! This practice makes a great game to play with a friend, to see who has the stronger Chi.

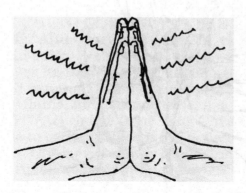

FOCUS EXERCISE - EYE PRACTICE

Next, from 3 feet away, focus your eyes on one end of the straw. With hands gently pressed together, in the praying position, just below your eye level, deeply breathe to your Chi Point. By gently drawing your Yin Chi from your eyes to your Chi Point, you should cause the end of the straw to pull toward you. Again, emphasize your inward breathing.

Next, forcefully press your hands together, and reverse the Chi from your Chi Point out your eyes, and cause the Yang Chi to push the straw away. Emphasize your outward breath, but do not breathe directly at the straw. Try the eye practice from various distances. Push or pull the straw with your eyes, by reversing your Chi flow.

This, too, takes a small mental effort. This is NOT black magic. This power is a gift from the Creator of the Universe and given to people who are created in His Image. It is NOT given to any other creature. It proves you are NOT an animal. Give God the thanks! (Note: Many first-time users fear the next exercise will cause harm to them. It will not! It is a vital exercise to practice if you are to control animals or birds. The highest medical authorities flatly state it causes no harm. The difficulty may be so great that you think you will become unconscious. Do it anyway! **You must master this exercise**!)

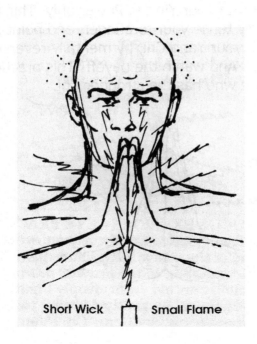

Short Wick   **Small Flame**

FOCUS EXERCISE - EXTINGUISH A CANDLE WITH YOUR EYES

As in PART II, fast tense your muscles in a wave from toes to fingertips, while standing. Again pump-build your Chi Power with hands tightly together in praying position. Use a standard household emergency candle. Birthday candles burn too quickly and will not be extinguished. Place the candle, with a very short wick and small flame, before you. Clip the wick to shorten it. Focus your eyes on the flame.

Now place your hands in the praying position at chest level, and press together very hard, while forcing the Yang Chi out of your eyes. Keep your gut very tight, while you slowly force-breathe into and out from your Chi Point. Don't breathe at the candle. Direct your outgoing breath toward your tensed gut. Your head may break out in a sweat. Watch the candle flame slowly die. With each of your Yang Chi, outgoing breaths, the flame becomes smaller until it goes out. This takes much effort and endurance. Beginners may wish to place the candle inside a pot lying on its side. DONT GIVE UP! (PRESS PAUSE BUTTON).

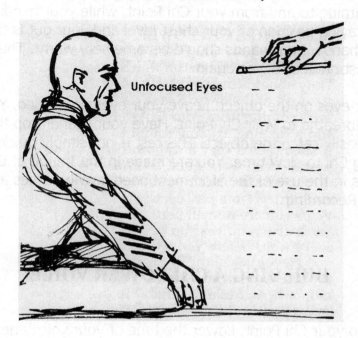

Unfocused Eyes

FOCUS EXERCISE - THROW YOUR YANG CHI TO EXTINGUISH THE FLAME

After you build your Chi, close one hand in a fist. From several feet away, open the other hand. With your fingers tightly cupped together, throw your Yang Chi at the candle flame. At the same time, use the YAH-HWAH Shout. Your Yang Chi should be able to extinguish the candle flame on impact. Chi moves slower than wind, so allow time for your Chi to reach the flame.

FOCUS EXERCISE - TIME CONTROL

Do not build your Chi. Sit cross-legged on the floor, hands at rest on your knees. Have a friend drop a pen or pencil at your arm's length away from you and at your eye level. Try to catch the object before it hits the ground or floor. Now build your Chi, by force-breathing to and from your Chi Point, while your hands are pressed together in the praying position at your chest level and your gut is tight. Direct your Yang Chi to your hands. Your hands should become very warm. Then place your warm hands at rest on your knees again.

Do not focus your eyes on the object. Leave your eyes unfocused. You must continue to force-breathe to your Chi Point. Have your friend drop the object again. You should now easily catch the object. This test is not simply quickened re-flexes. This is using Yang Chi to slow time. You are made in the Image of God, Creator of Time. The proof is in the use of the aforementioned gravity forces and it can save your life! (End of Recording.)

BUILDING A CHI POWER VOICE

Deeply breathe to your Chi Point. Lower the tone of your voice and force the words you speak. They should come out from your throat strongly and slowly. Speak as if your voice were coming from your Chi Point. Try to add a rasping, cutting sound to your voice. It should be a very low, powerful, rasping sound. Each word must be forced from your throat with as much power as you can muster. As time passes, the Chi Power Voice you create will become a habit.

This habit also requires you to think strongly of every word before you speak it. Never use slang or curse words! Words are like two-edged swords. They can wound, kill, or heal. Make it a habit to use words that ennoble the person or creature to whom you speak. If you don't understand the exact meaning of words, use a dictionary to learn them. Almost all English words have several meanings. It is extremely important to know the exact meaning of the word you wish to speak or write.

There are small hand-size computer-type dictionaries with a thesaurus of words that have the same meaning. A dictionary should be your constant companion for quick reference. Voice communication is the most important skill you will ever learn. While you are learning the Chi Power Voice, you will be gaining self respect. It was by words that worlds were created and angels fell. Treat words with extreme respect, and respect will be given you by others that will humble you. Pride and learning are incompatable.

A proud person cannot learn. A humble person is willing to listen, and learns much. Again we caution you to use the Chi Power Voice with extreme care. Do not hurt others with it except under extreme provocation.

PROBLEM SOLVING

If you have trouble getting things to work, ask a friend to help you. **EVERYTHING WORKS EXACTLY AS STATED**. Don't give up.

Static electricity in a very dry room can void your Chi. It may help to boil water, to add moisture to the room. Also, anxiety drugs or sleeping pills can void your Chi Power. Regular use of prescription or nonprescription drugs can shrink your blood vessels to the point of causing great weakness. You may have Yin Chi, but your Yang Chi will usually be very weak. More than that, your glandular system will be unbalanced. Regular Chi Power practice can help restore the size of your blood vessels, and balance your internal organs.

If you are directing Chi to pull or push a straw, wipe the straw with a dry cloth first, to remove dust and ion pollution. Over breathing (too fast breathing) can cause hyperventilation, with undesirable symptoms. Simply hold your breath and run in place, or pump your arms, for the symptoms to disappear. (Or breathe into a bag.) Then correct your breathing by slowing the number of breaths per minute. You probably will have to repeat the tensing process.

WEIGHT-LIFTERS

Because you have very large blood vessels caused by every day practice, you may have a bit of difficulty when first trying to build your Chi. We suggest you limit your weight--lifting to three times per week.

SAMPLE CHI POWER PLUS PROGRAM

1. LIGHT STRETCHING - Start gently stretching and loosening up your muscles and joints. No maximum stretching unless your body is sweating. Spend about five minutes on this exercise.

2. LIGHT SLAPPING EXERCISE -Start slapping or hitting all of your body surface areas with the palms of your hands, concentrating especially around the inside of each elbow, back of each knee, kidney area, up and down each armpit, and on your thymus area (refer to Chi Chart for loca-. tions). By slapping lightly on each of these areas, you will open up the skin pores and stimulate your nerve fibers more effectively. Spend 60-90 seconds on this exercise.

3. BLOOD WASHING / SENSITIVITY TRAINING EXERCISE - Learn to perform this exercise regularly, as it will greatly increase your Chi by making your nerve fibers bigger and stronger. The exercise also helps your body maintain a stronger polar-ity. Refer to the handout sheet provided, in order to learn the exercise. Spend 3-5 mins on this exercise.

4. PROVIDED TAPE EXERCISES:
a) 3-MIN LUNG BUILDING EXERCISE - Really try to push yourself, since you're only doing this exercise for three mins. Try to inhale and exhale as long and as slowly as you can, breathing through your mouth only to begin with. You will be able to open up your lower lung system easier and quicker, by using your mouth instead of your nose for the first couple of months practice.

b) TENSE / RELAX & ORGAN BALANCE EXERCISES - Perform these exercises like on the tape. If you do just the exercises only, it takes about 15 mins.
5. STANDING MEDITATION-Learn to perform this exercise on a daily basis m order to build strong Yang Chi. Refer to the "How To Start Your Chi Program" sheets, Page 3, to learn this exercise. After you can do this exercise for at least 10 mins, start performing the Bone Marrow / Energy Pack-ing Exercise while doing your standing meditation exercise (refer to handout sheet in order to perform this exercise). Beginners spend five or more minutes. Advanced spend from 20-60 mins. This is a hard exercise, but if you train your body to perform this exer-cise every day, you will find that it will get easier to perform, over time. Learn to relax your body, even though it wants to tighten; try to disassociate yourself from the pain while performing this exercise. Also, don't stare at a clock while doing this exercise, but close your eyes and you will be able to do it longer; or you can even perform this exercise while playing music or watching TV in order to disassociate yourself from the pain in your feet and legs. The pain you feel at first will go away in time as you are able to train your body to handle this type of exercise.

6. FINISHING EXERCISE - Finish up your exercise routine by performing the Blood Washing / Sensitivity Exercise again. Perform the Palm Test to see how strong your Chi is, after doing the Chi exercises (refer to Page 6 of "How to Start Your Chi Program" sheets).

CHI POWER TIPS

Concentrate on performing the exercises with quality rather than quantity for better results. Perform the exercises daily (not only three times a week) for fastest results. All the exercises will become easier to perform over time as you make them a habit. Your Chi power will also be enhanced by providing your body with proper diet/nutrition and by taking vitamin, mineral and herb supplements.

FOCUS TESTS: Try practicing putting out the candle or moving the straw exercises using both methods, as explained in the Chi Power Plus Booklet (Yang Chi/Yang Style) or in the "How To Start Your Chi Power Plus Program", Pages 5 & 6 (Yang Chi/Yin Style). See which method is easier for you to perform and use that way. Don't use the hanging straw for yang throws. Put up some other type of hanging object in order to work on getting your throws down. Practicing regularly on creating the steady flow of Chi helps you to create a better yang throw.

ADDITIONAL CHI TECHNIQUES: VARIATION #I OF PALM TEST: Try doing the Palm Test (refer to Page 6 of "How to Start your Chi Program") with this variation: Since the Chi energy will go through practically anything you send it through, stand m a doorway and put one hand on one side of the wall and your other hand on the other side of the wall. Do not touch the wall, but leave a 5 - 10 inch gap between your palms and the wall. Now do the Palm Test. You will find that you can feel the Chi energy go right through the wall.

VARIATION #2 OF PALM TEST; This time, while you. do the Palm Test, have someone put his or her hand into the space between your palms, so that they feel the energy pass through their hand. Practice sending the Chi energy through an object, as well as stopping it at or within an object.

REGARDING SIDE EFFECTS

The exercises we have included in the SPC-USA Chi Power Plus program should cause you no bad side effects. Some Chi programs available elsewhere can cause side effects. If you plan to study other Chi courses along with our program, be sure you have opened the Chi channels in your arms and legs first. Be absolutely certain you have done this before working on methods which take Chi energy straight up to your head, or you will definitely experience side effects. When you stimulate any part of your body, it is done by an electrical pulse which travels back and forth from the brain to the part stimulated, using nerve fibers in your body to send the message. If too much electrical energy is sent through a nerve fiber before it is prepared to handle it, it can cause an overload and possible damage. Learn to develop and strengthen your nerve fibers by doing our exercises regularly (especially the Blood Washing Exercise). If on any day, you do not have time to do all the SPC-USA Chi exercises, be sure you get the Night Exercises/Yin Time done.

NIGHT EXERCISES/YIN TIME

1. LIGHT STRETCHING - Do some light stretching before going to bed. Spend 3' 5 minutes.

2. BLOOD WASHING / SENSITIVITY TRAINING - Perform this exercise just before getting into bed. Spend 3-4 mins on exercise.

3. LYING DOWN MEDITATION EXERCISE - Perform this exercise in your bed (refer to Page 4 of "How To Start Your Chi Program"). Your attracting power (Yin Chi) will increase with. regular practice of this exercise. Beginners spend 15-20 mins. Advanced perform tills exercise from 30-60 mins.

Version 2.0

Getting Started With Chi Power Training

First, you. need to read the Chi Power Plus booklet and the chi info sheets included in your package. Then listen to the audio tape, which includes info on building a Chi Power voice. You do not need to read the Prolepsis booklet at this time ("prolepsis" means "a story of how it could have been"). The Prolepsis does not include any information on how to build your chi.

Read everything about building the chi more than once for those areas that interest you the most. It is very easy to read over important information, so reading it at least several times will help you avoid missing anything.

You don't have to be a martial artist, or even an athlete, to learn how to do the chi. You only need determination to learn.

Chi energy can be expelled from your body as a quick surge (for throwing or breaking) or as a steady stream of ions (for manipulating objects or living things). To externalize strong chi, of either type, you must first increase your lung capacity.

LEARN TO DEEP BREATHE

To begin with, you must get the breathing down right. There are three different breathing exercises you need to learn to get the chi to work. The three types are (1) chi gung (also called chi kung) or relaxed deep breathing, with long inhale and long exhale, (2) yang chi rhythm, with long exhale and short inhale, and (3) yin chi rhythm, with long inhale and short exhale. Chi gung breathing will be used when going through the tape exercises and when you do any type of meditation. Yang rhythm is used to repel things and yin rhythm is used to attract.

Chi gung breathing is done by allowing yourself to relax and taking a long inhale (making your inhale longer than your normal breathing, by slowly letting your lungs expand and controlling the air flow), then slowly exhaling (making your exhale longer than your normal exhale, again by controlling the air flow). Be sure you are breathing deep enough that your abdomen expands on the inhale and contracts on the exhale.

Chi gung breathing is done slowly and relaxed. If you find you are getting dizzy or feeling light-headed after several breaths, you need to slow down your breathing pattern. Chi gung breathing can be done through either your nose or mouth (most people practice this type in through the nose and out through the mouth). We want you to practice breathing through your mouth to ~ begin with, in order to get the other two types of breathing rhythm down easier. After several months of practice you will be able to create the energy through either your nose or mouth.

YANG CHI RHYTHM

To create the yang chi rhythm, which is used to repel things, you need to make a short inhale (still deep breathing) and then a long exhale through your mouth. Your inhale should only last one to two seconds, and the exhale should last at least five to ten seconds. As you get better at doing the breathing exercises, your exhale breath will last longer (a good exhale of 15 to 30 seconds will give you better control). To make sure you are doing it properly, place your hand in front of your mouth a few inches away. When you exhale, make an audible noise (sub-vocal sound) trying to get it to come

from as deep in your throat as possible. Your mouth should be slightly open in an oval shape, and you want to use the "hahhhhhh" sound. When you exhale you should only feel a little bit of air on your hand. If you feel a lot of air, you need to practice making it only a little. Again, if you find that after several breaths, you are getting dizzy or light- headed then you are breathing too fast. When you slow down your breathing your dizziness will go away. As you are able to control your vocal cords in your throat, you will get a better pattern of breathing without the fluctuation that occurs when you are first learning.

YIN CHI RHYTHM

To create the yin chi rhythm, which attracts things, you do the exact opposite of the yang chi. You want to inhale making the same audible noise (the "hahhhhhh" sound) through your mouth. You should try to make your inhale (still deep breathing) last as long as you can and then exhale for only a second or two.

Make sure you are actually taking in air flow and not just making the sound - your lungs will slowly fill up (first the bottom, then the top) as you are inhaling. When you first start doing this type of breathing it will feel a little uncomfortable; but as you continue to practice, it will be- come easier to do. We recommend that you practice the breathing (yin and yang rhythm) nine to ten times throughout the day for several minutes at a time, so your body gets used to the exercise, and it becomes easier to do. It usually takes a week or so of practicing the breathing exercises to become proficient at them.

ON THE AUDIO

You should try to use the tape provided, and go through each of the exercises once a day. If you find this tape goes too fast or slow for you to comfortably use, record your own tape (instructions are in the booklet). Usually the tape provided will work if the announcer's heartbeat is close to the same as yours.

The chi gung breathing exercise (Part I on the tape and in the booklet), where you put a weight (such as a book, or even a magazine) on your abdomen and practice for three minutes is designed to teach you to breathe from your lower, as well as upper, lung system.

This increases your lung capacity, so you will be able to breathe much longer inhales and exhales. This will help you create a better chi rhythm. By chi rhythm, we mean doing your breaths the same way every time, so that you create a steady flow of ions. You are doing the exercise right when you can go to the very end of your breath without gasping. Then when you're practicing the chi gung breathing in the other exercises, or while meditating, you won't be going to the end of your breath, but about 50% to 75% of it.

PART II - TENSION EXERCISES

The tension exercises are designed to help you individualize your joints and muscles, so they work independently from each other. We know that when the tape says to tighten up your right toe, your whole leg will most likely tighten. If you practice regularly, learning to concentrate on only the part of the body we're talking about, you will find that you will be able to tighten up only your foot instead of your whole leg; or only your hand instead of your whole arm and chest. You will find that these exercises will really improve your speed with regular practice. This is because the tendons and muscles in your arm or leg won't be slowing you down while throwing a punch or kick, as they do when they're in a constricted state. Remember that a relaxed body is much faster than a tight one. During the tension exercise, you should be breathing rhythmically (chi gung breathing) the same amount in as you are out.

Because many of you are anxious to see something happen, the tape tells you to move to your practice hanging object and throw your chi at it. Do not use the straw for throwing your chi - you need the straw for learning to use the yang and yin chi for manipulation.

PART III - ORGAN BALANCING EXERCISES

The next set of exercises is designed to keep your organs in good working condition.

To do these exercises properly, you want to tighten up your hand and place it on the organ (use the poster provided in order to know where to put your hand). You should concentrate on and visualize each organ while breathing in an even inhale and exhale type chi gung rhythm. While inhaling try to imagine the energy flowing out from the organ and into your hand. When you exhale, try to imagine the energy flowing from your hand into the organ. With practice you will find that your hand will warm up and you will actually feel this energy flow. Normally, you will feel the energy leave your hand and go into the organ on the exhale, after you have been practicing a while (usually after a week or two).

Feeling the energy leaving your organ and going into your hand on the inhale normally takes a lot longer. With practice you will be able to feel the energy flow in both directions. As you train your body to be more sensitive, the energy will become stronger.

It's very important that you go through this part even if you think you're in great shape physically. It will help insure that you stay that way. For the organs to function well, they need as much blood flow as possible. Even if one of the organs has been removed, still cover it, since it will help protect the cavity from disease. The statements you repeat either out loud or to yourself are designed to improve your mental attitude. Externalizing chi requires mental as well as physical effort.

PART IV - SLOW MOVING RELAXATION EXERCISES

Part IV goes through the relaxation (slow moving meditation). This exercise was designed to help your circulation and energy flow. This exercise is shown from an advanced form, where you are sitting in a crossed legs (lotus position) fashion. If you find this position too uncomfortable, lie flat on your back with your knees bent. or sit in a chair. The important thing is that you get your body to completely relax during the exercise. To do this, you need to let your arms and legs go completely limp, so that you take all movement out of them. If you

find that any part of your body doesn't want to relax, try tightening that part and then relaxing it. Concentrate on the energy flow. The tension exercises constrict your artery flow and the relaxation exercises help to enlarge them. Your chi flow will increase with practice. This is an important part of the program. Learning to both constrict and enlarge your arteries helps keep them flexible, to keep you in a healthy state of being. It will also help keep your arteries clear of plaque buildup which causes hardening of the arteries.

MEDITATION TECHNIQUES

The next two types of meditations (standing and lying down) can be practiced after going through the tape exercises. The standing meditation used in conjunction with the lying down meditation will provide you with the fastest method possible for building your chi energy stronger. If you find the standing meditation too hard to do at first, practice doing the slow moving and lying down meditation exercises daily for awhile, and slowly add the standing meditation exercise into your chi building routine.

STANDING MEDITATION

The standing meditation exercise is the hardest to perform, but is also the quickest way to build strong yang chi. You perform this exercise by standing in a horse stance if you are familiar with martial arts terminology or by standing with your feet a little farther apart than shoulder width. You should have only a slight bend in your knees if you are just learning to do this type of exercise. Hold your arms out like you were carrying a basket of apples, but don't interlock your fingers. There should be at least a five to ten inch distance between your hands and you should spread your fingers (keep a slight gap in between each finger).

Keep your elbows close in to your sides, as this will allow you to do the exercise longer without as much pain or strain on your back. You should keep your back straight and your head looking straight ahead not looking toward the ground. As your body gets used to doing this exercise itwill get a little easier to perform. If you. are just beginning this type of exercise, try to stand in this position for five minutes in the morning and five minutes at night.

When you can perform this exercise for the whole five minutes for a full week, you should start adding a minute a day until you can perform the standing exercise for thirty minutes.

Some people perform this exercise for a whole hour or longer, and are able to build huge amounts of energy. It takes most people several months of practice to get to this level.

While doing this standing meditation try to concentrate on chi gung breathing. During your inhale try to visualize yourself sucking up energy off the ground and make the energy travel up your legs and into your chi point. You should breathe through your nose on the inhale and out your mouth with the exhale. It normally takes several weeks of practice before you are literally able to feel this energy flow pattern traveling up your legs.
On your exhale (while chi gung breathing), you should switch your concentration to your fingertips. While exhaling mentally feel the energy shooting out your fingertips. At first, your fingertips will heat up and later you will start feeling the heat energy coming out your fingertips. The energy will feel like a magnetic field wave coming from. your fingers.

To make a smaller-in-diameter energy laser beam (electrical-magnetic field wave) shoot out your index finger, you should practice doing the standing meditation with only your two index fingers pointing at each other with at least a 3-4 inch gap between them, with the rest of your hand closed into a fist. This will allow you to put out the candle easier.

To create a much wider energy laser beam shooting from your hands, all you need to do is turn your hands so that more of your palm is showing toward each other and concentrate on the heat energy going out the palms of your hands. People normally practice this method to build their healing power techniques. Used with acupressure, this type of healing method can be used for deeper penetration to the sore areas of the body. Also practicing the meditation, with your arms out *from* your body with the palms of your hands facing toward the ground will help you build a larger energy field wave.

When you first start doing the standing meditation, your body may begin to sweat (sometimes a little and sometimes a lot). This is normal as your body gets rid of toxins which have built up in the body. Your body may shake or tremble when you first start doing the exercise. This will change as you are able to relax your body even though it is in a state of tension from the exercise.

As you learn to hold the stance longer and longer, you normally will feel different strange sensations happening inside your body. As you open up your chi channels (which simply means your blood flow is better), you will feel a stronger energy field wave. As you learn to externalize your chi, you will sweat less as the energy used by the body to sweat will be used to build a stronger field wave. Simply learning to mentally concentrate on the energy flow and less on your body pain allows this process to take place.

You use this standing meditation method to build your yang (repelling) chi stronger when using it for a steady flow of energy. You can use the pump build method on Page 25 of the Chi Power Plus booklet (and on the tape) if you want to build a surge of chi quickly for yang throws or breaks.

LYING DOWN MEDITATION

You should get into a comfortable position where you are lying flat on your back on your bed, with your arms out from your body at a 45 degree angle. The palms of your hands should be down on the bed. For the first few minutes take even breaths in and out that are slow and relaxing (chi gung breathing). After that, taper of ton your breathing so that you are barely breathing in and out. Just like on the tape get each part of your body to relax. Next, concentrate on each of your toes and fingers. Start in a clockwise direction and mentally feel each individual finger and toe, starting with your left hand, going to your left foot, then right

foot and right hand. You should be able to mentally feel each finger and toe without moving them; if you can't at first, then make the smallest amount of movement possible, in order to be able to feel them.

As you practice doing this exercise, it will become easier and easier to feel the energy. It will feel like a tingling sensation at first and after awhile you should be able to feel the pulse rate in each finger and toe. This helps to enlarge your arteries. Spend five seconds mentally concentrating on each individual finger and toe. After going through five total clockwise rotations, you should be able to feel a good energy flow. Remain on your bed in this position for about 25-30 minutes. The rest of the time can be used for moving the chi to different parts and on learning to open your third eye.

You may at first feel a little stiff or find that your body may twitch here and there, but these symptoms will go away with a little practice. You will find that this lying down meditation will be very effective in helping you to build yin (attracting) chi..

If you have been doing a lot of weight lifting, or other muscle building exercises, you may need to spend a considerable amount of time practicing the lying down meditation and the blood-washing exercise before you can see any results from the rest of the program.

VISIONS

Normally you will go through several stages of relaxation before you are able to see visions through your third eye (the white area between your eyes like on the poster). In the first stage you aren't relaxed enough, so all you feel is some tingling sensations here and there. In the second stage, you may see different colors or negative images. You may also feel like you're floating on air or have some other type of strange sensation. The third stage, where you are really able to get into a deep state of relaxation, will open the door for visions. Even in the third stage you will not see visions every time.

A true vision is God's message especially for you and He is the one who will reveal its meaning, sometimes even months later. Don't be discouraged if you can't reach this level of competence right away as it takes some people longer than others to do and has a lot to do with how much stress you have in your life. As with all the techniques you are learning, the more you practice the better and easier they become.

CHI AS A SURGE OF ENERGY

The chi energy works as a surge of energy or as a steady flow. To make a surge of chi all you do is make a quick inhale and quick exhale. You will find that using the Joshua shout, where you make the "yah" sound as you quickly inhale and the "whah" sound as you quickly exhale, will give you a great deal of power with practice. For a yang chi throw or break, it is important to get the timing down, so that your exhale and flip of the wrist for the throw is at the same time. For breaks, the contact to the board or brick should be made at the same time as your exhale breath for best results. The circular motion (or partially rounded movements) we are talking about when doing a yang throw can be done two ways. One way is to make the throw like a ridge-hand throw in karate or like throwing a discus in gymnastics. The second way is to make the throw like you were throwing shurikens (throwing stars) or a frisbee. Make sure you flip your wrist with the exhale. Your concentration must be on the target. With practice you will find you can get farther and farther away from an object and still hit it.

CHI AS A STEADY FLOW OF ENERGY

For manipulating, you need a steady flow of chi. To move the straw away from you or to put the candle out (yang chi), you must make a lot longer exhale than inhale. Make sure your breathing is slow and relaxed, and that you are not tensing up the wrong part of your body. In other words, if you are tensing your feet as you try to move the straw, all your chi energy will go down to your feet, and you won't be able to move the straw.

 Also make sure you are concentrating on the straw (about an inch from the end of it) or the wick if looking at the candle. Don't concentrate on tightening your chi point or gut, as it will happen naturally when you are doing the breathing right (if you concentrate on your chi point the energy will come out there or simply stay there). As you get better and are able to create more chi energy you will find that you will not have to tense up your body or use as much energy getting the chi to flow out of you.

The candle exercise may make you break out in a sweat when you first try it, but with practice it will become easier to do and take a lot less concentration. Try cutting the wick of the candle down as much as possible (until it almost goes out by itself). When you are able to get it out like that, you can let the wick get longer and longer until you don't need to cut it down anymore. Then to make it harder, try to get farther and farther away from the candle and still be able to get it to go out.

You will find practicing your standing meditation using the index finger only method will enhance your ability to put out the candle, since this will allow your body to put off a smaller in diameter field wave. Practice putting the candle out by using either your eyes or your index finger.

When you inhale, your body puts off more negative ions than positive ones, which causes things to be attracted to you. To get the straw to come to you, breathe yin chi. Make your inhale much longer than your exhale. Deep breathe slowly and relaxed. Point your finger at the end of the straw you want to come toward you, take a long slow inhale, and think in your mind you want the end of the straw to turn toward you. Remember that your focus must be on where you want the chi to go.

PALM TEST EXERCISE

One way to check on how much chi you have right now is to do this exercise. Sit or stand, putting your hands in a praying position (where the palms of your hands are right against each other). Next, spread your hands apart about 10 to 15 inches, keeping them parallel or horizontal with each other. Slowly move your hands an inch or two toward each other, then an inch or two away from each other. Slowly repeat several times. Concentrate on the palms of your hands. You should be able to mentally feel the palms without physically touching them. You should feel a slight tingling or magnetic

type energy flowing from one palm to the other. You may feel this energy right away or through practice be able to develop it. Most people will be able to feel it the first time they try the exercise. If you have a hard time feeling the energy, start by concentrating on one palm at a time, feeling the air touching the palm. There's usually at least 20 degrees difference between your body temperature and the air in the room, so with just a little bit of concentration, you should feel the air. Then concentrate on feeling the energy flow from palm to palm. You will find that with a little practice, you will be able to still feel this energy flow even though you spread your hands out farther and farther away from each other. Try this Palm Test before and after you go through the chi exercises, and you will see a big difference.

A TYPICAL CHI PROGRAM

A typical chi program consists of: stretching and warm up exercises, going through the blood washing/sensitivity exercise, listening and going through the provided tape (or one that you have recorded with just the exercises on them), performing the meditation exercises and working on some of the chi exercises like the straw or candle, etc. Then practice your own style of conditioning exercises or martial arts for whatever style you enjoy doing (or practicing yoga, katas, aerobics, etc.). Beginners normally spend 45 minutes daily doing the chi exercises, and later extend the time to an hour or 90 minutes as they train their body to handle it.

PLEASE NOTE:

We've added this information to your package to further explain some of the important points of the program, and to cover the most frequently asked questions. If you still have questions or problems, please write, or call when you can talk to an instructor, Monday thru Friday, noon till 8 pm Eastern Time Zone.

Blood Washing/Sensitivity Training

This exercise should be performed three times daily. It only takes a couple of minutes to do and. over time will really help improve your chi. Perform the exercise when you first get up and just before going to bed. The third time is done before going through the recorded chi tape exercises. The exercise is designed to stimulate all your surface skin nerve endings on your arms and legs, so that better communication between your brain and the individual joint, muscle, or tendon will take place.

The more you stimulate an area the stronger you make the communicative pathway. Your nerves control the small muscles that surround the arteries which help control the blood flow. By physically stimulating your skin nerve endings, you make them more sensitive. The more sensitive you make the areas, the easier it is to mentally feel that area. The daily practice of this exercise will help sensitize your body.

To perform this exercise you can either sit or stand. Take your right hand (palm down) and put it on your left shoulder. Start lightly rubbing down the outside of your left arm (rubbing slowly, touching all the skin surface area) until you reach your fingertips. At the fingertips, slightly squeeze the tips of each finger and thumb.

Then start rubbing up the inside of your left arm to the armpit. Next, rub down. from the left armpit, down the left side, down the outside of the left leg, until you get to the foot. At the foot, you should rub the entire foot area and slightly pinch each toe tip. Then, rub up the inside of the left leg to the groin.

At the groin you change hands, Starting with your left hand, rub down the inside of your right leg to the foot. Rub your entire right foot and slightly pinch each toe. Rub up the outside of the right leg, up the right side till you reach your armpit. Next, rub down the inside of your right arm to the fingertips. Slightly pinch each fingertip and thumb.

Rub up the outside of the hand, up the outside of the arm to the right shoulder. This process should be done three times m the same clockwise method each time you perform the exercise.

Perform this exercise as described for two weeks. After two weeks, start adding into this exercise the following variation. When you get to the part where you are ending your third rota- tion of rubbing around your body, you should change to doing the fourth rotation like this: Instead of actually resting your hand on your left shoulder, start with your right hand about an inch or two above the surface skin of the shoulder.

Perform the exercise just as before, except you are not making actual skin contact this time. Even as you get to the part where you . gently squeeze your fingertips or toe tips, you don't want to actually make contact, but still go through the process. Do a fifth and sixth rotation.

Then complete the exercise by putting both hands above your head so that your fingertips are almost touching. Your palms should be facing toward the top of your head, but should be three to four inches above the skin surface of your head. Next bring your hands slowly down the front of your body (not making contact) until you reach your chi point. You should start your inhale as your hands leave your head area, and finish the inhale as your hands stop at your chi point. You should exhale into your chi point, then tighten up your whole body for a second just as you finish your exhale.

With time you will feel your chi actually stimulating and bouncing off your skin surface, even though you are not making contact.

This exercise will also help your chi circulate better throughout your body, and keep you properly polarized (maintaining a better positive and negative ion flow).

When you first start, you might want to perform this exercise with only your shorts on. With. practice you can feel the energy with or without clothing being there.

Bone Marrow Energy Packing

This is an advanced exercise to be per- formed only after you are able to externalize your chi. You should be able to at least move the straw around (while it is hanging from the string) in either direction or at least feel a fair amount of heat energy coming from the palms of your hands when you do the Palm Test Exercise in "How To Start Your Chi Power Plus Program". This exercise should be performed right after you do the "Blood Washing/Sensitivity Training". It will help considerably if you can do the exercise near live plants or trees.

PART 1:

Begin by sitting on a bench or the side of a bed (later on, you'll probably prefer standing). Start the exercise by bending over and reaching down with your hands and arms toward your feet. Keep the palms of your hands turned in toward your body, with at least a 5-6 inch gap between your palms and your legs. Get a mental picture or image of your hands acting like vacuum cleaners sucking up energy off the ground around your feet. Reach your hands out, with your fingers spread wide, and gather in the energy. Slowly lift your hands up your legs toward your chi point area, as you take a long relaxed inhale thru your nose. Your body and hands should be relaxed. As you lift your hands, think of the energy spiraling up your legs and into your chi point.

Next, start packing the chi energy into your organs like you would pack snow on a snowman, as you make a long relaxed exhale through your mouth. You are not actually making contact with your body, but keeping your palms at least 5-6 inches from your body as you pack. Your palms should be cupped tensely so you can pack in a lot of energy. Pack in the chi energy for 15-20

seconds, covering all your lower organ areas and the pelvic area (front and back). Then, move up to your lungs and neck and continue to pack for another 10-15 seconds. If needed, take a quick inhale of air before you continue to the chest and neck. Again start slowly exhaling as you pack. Next) reach down and grab more energy and again start the packing process. You should perform this exercise for at least three or four minutes at a time.

PART 2:

When you have practiced Part I enough times that you can strongly feel the chi travel up your legs, you're ready to add Part 2. Reach down and grab more energy, and while slowly exhaling, pack it into each arm and into each leg. Remember that you don't touch the surface. After you exhale and before you inhale, tighten up your body to squeeze and condense the energy in. Be sure you are thinking of the bone area you want the chi to condense into. Do as many grabs with inhale) and packs with exhale, as it takes to cover the entire length of your arms and legs.

To finish the exercise, whether you're doing only Part I or both parts, you should do three more Blood Washing rotations where you rub down your body without actually touching the skin.

Even if you have not built up enough lung capacity to inhale for 10-15 seconds or exhale for 30 seconds, you can still do the exercise. With practice, your lungs will expand, allowing you longer breaths. When you regularly perform this exercise, your chi power, along with your ability to externalize it, will increase substantially.

"INNER CIRCLE" & "CLOSED DOOR"

MASTER SECRETS of Qigong &

CHI POWER

Secret trainings and techniques that until now have never been shared with anyone other than our closest, most personal students

Scientific Premium Company- USA

Introduction

What is the Inner Circle?

The *Inner Circle* is an online community where men and women interested in cultivating and growing their knowledge, awareness, and understanding of *chi* can receive detailed instructions from Masters who have gone before them. Students receive consultation and training techniques/exercises specifically tailored to their level of progression.

Conference calls between the Master Instructors and interviews with Instructor who have trained with the Masters along with accompanying articles are available for review via the Inner Circle website. There, members of the Inner Circle have access to a wealth of knowledge, gleaned from the past successes and pitfalls of those who have gone before them.

What is behind the Closed Door?

The *Closed Door* is a system designed to take members who have completed the training regimen offered in the Inner Circle to the next level of chi ability. The Closed Door system is a much more involved training environment, where the margin of error grows slimmer and slimmer the more your chi energy increases; although many want to gain access into the Closed Door System, only a very select few, handpicked by the Master Instructors will be invited into said community. High moral values and a steadfast mind are needed more than ever when entering chi development/cultivation at this level.

Many are called, few are chosen...

"INNER CIRCLE" & "CLOSED DOOR" **54**

Secret trainings and techniques that until now have never been shared with anyone other than our closest, most personal students 54

Scientific Premium Company- USA **54**

Introduction **55**
    What is the Inner Circle? **55**
    What is behind the Closed Door? **55**

Chapter 1: What is Chi? **59**
    The Physics behind the Mysticism **59**
        Chi and the Human Body 59

        Chi and the Brain 59

    Electricity & Chi: One and the Same **62**
        Bioelectricity 62

        Bioelectricity and the Body 63

        Chi and the Body Continued 64

    Chi, the Inner Circle, and You! **64**

Chapter 2: The SPC Method **65**
    Mental Preparation **65**
        Ascending Euphoria 65

        Affirmations and Autosuggestion 65

    Chi Distillation **66**
    Physical Exercises **66**
        Bloodwashing 66

        Standing Meditation 66

        Lying Down Meditation 67

        Micro/Macro Cosmic Orbits [month 3] 67

Chapter 3: The Inner Circle **68**
    Welcome **68**
    About the IC **68**
    The Nature of Chi **68**
        Circular Chi vs. Linear Chi 68

Three Stages of Chi.. 69

Light Chi & Heavy Chi.. 70

Nutrition and Chi Power... **71**

Chapter 4: Inner Circle Curriculum **72**

Techniques and Building Blocks **72**

Telekinesis and Psi abilities **72**

Using Chi to Bend Metal 72

Got Skills?... 73

Sensing Objects... 73

Sensing Colors 73

OBE 74

Remote Viewing & Astral Projection.................................. 74

Advanced Healing Techniques 75

Transferring Energy: Hot and Cold Temperatures 75

The Law of Attraction.. **76**

Pheromones **76**

Pheromones: "Yin and Yang".. 77

Pheromones and Chi 77

Pheromones and the Inner Circle.. 78

Emotional Content.. **78**

Chi Training Partner **80**

Chapter 5: Inner Circle Community **81**

Questions & Answers Sessions and Topics **81**

Q & A Session 1 81

Q & A Session 2 83

Q & A Session 3 83

Q & A Session 4 85

Q & A Session 5 86

Q & A Session 6 88

Q & A Session 7 90

Q & A Session 8 92

    Q & A Session 9 94

Interviews with Certified Instructors 96
    Sifu Michael Allen.. 96

    Sifu Benjamin Richardson 96

    Sifu Andrei Biesinger 98

    Sifu Charles Dragoo... 98

    Sifu Don Brown 98

Chapter 6: The Closed Door................................... 99
    Behind the Closed Door 99
    Two 6 Month Intensive Training System 99
    The 1st 6 Months (Form Chi) 99
    Closed Door: Module One (Release of Advanced Chi DVD Volume 3)   100
    Closed Door: ModuleTwo (Body Breathing) 100
    Closed Door: Module Three (Advanced OBE) 100
    Closed Door: Module Four (Wall to Wall Exercise) 100
    Closed Door: Module Five (Advanced Circle Training).......... 100
    Closed Door: Module Six (Levitation 101) 101
    The 2nd 6 Months Closed Door System (Super Set 101
    Training).. 101
    Closed Door: Module Seven (Effective Control Methods) 101
    Closed Door: Module Eight (Liquid Chi).................... 101
    Closed Door: Module Nine (Hypnotic Devices Training) 101
    Closed Door: Module Ten (Super Set Variations).................. 102
    Closed Door: Module Eleven (Fractal Images)....................... 102
    Closed Door: Module Twelve (Integration of All Techiques) . 102

Scientific Premium Company-USA Products 103
    Chi Power Plus... 103

    Advanced Chi Training System 103

Mind Force Collection of Esoteric Products 103

Chapter 1: What is Chi?

The Physics behind the Mysticism

Although surrounded by ancient mysticism, chi is that which Western scientists have called the Quantum Field. The theories are markedly similar when compared side-by-side. Each [Chinese Mysticism and Quantum Mechanics[1]] speaks of an energy field made up of tiny particles that comprise everything, and move through everything.

Looking at it from a scientific point of view, the shroud of mystery is removed, and an objective, scientific perspective remains

Chi and the Human Body

With the understanding that chi, synonymous with quantum particles, makes up everything and moves through every object, it logically extends that human beings are also made up of these small particles and as both camps postulate, this energy moves through everything.

In the movie, the Matrix, it is proposed that:

"The human body generates more bio-electricity than a 120-volt battery and over 25,000 BTUs of body heat"

This is a form of energy.

"According to the Center for Space Power and Advanced Electronics, a NASA commercial center in Alabama, the human body is capable of producing 11,000 watt hours. Broken into usable terms, waiting to be harvested are 81 watts from a sleeping person, 128 from a soldier standing at ease, 163 from a walking person, 407 from a briskly walking person, 1,048 from a long-distance runner, and 1,630 from a sprinter, according to the center. "[2]

When explaining chi to friends, I like to do a simple example that many people can perform.

Place your index finger in the air; wiggle it. This is a rudimentary example of electricity in motion; more specifically, bio-electromagnetic energy, in motion.

The brain sends an electric signal through the nervous system that reaches the finger, informing it to wiggle as your thoughts suggested. These electrical impulses that the body produces are manifestations of quantum mechanics: chi. Extending this analogy, we can view the nervous system as a bio-electromagnetic circuit; this has huge implications with regards to the SPC USA exercises, such as blood-washings, which we will speak to in separate articles in appropriate depth and detail.

Chi and the Brain

The human brain is quite possibly the most advanced system on planet Earth. We at SPC USA view it as a system because, when viewed as a singular component in the complex structure called the human body, the human brain itself is composed of many

---

[1] Quantum mechanics is the study of how the tiny particles which make up atoms behave
[2] http://www.space.com/businesstechnology/technology/body_power_011128-1.html

http://www.ChiPowerInnerCircle.com

differing components working together to perform to the various functions of what we have come to call the physical "brain".

At SPC-USA, we have studied how the brain works as well as how the brain functions; and use the most appropriate and safeguarded techniques when dealing with this intricate and delicate organ while using chi energy. We are very specific with the information you need to know to effectively, and safely, send energy through any of the brain areas.

The human brain is, in fact, as system of systems, that is: the brain is a system composed of multiple, independent systems. Within the brain we find: the limbic system, which regulates our hormones and emotions; the nervous system [of which the brain is the controlling agent of the nerves and nerve fiber running through the body]; as well as various hemispheres through which various functions are attributed- akin to the division of labor in an automobile factory.

Scientific advances over the course of time have contributed to our understanding of the brain: Magnetic Resonance Imaging (MRI) and Functional MRI (fMRI); Computed Axial Topography (CAT) Scans; Positron Emission Tomography (PET); as well as a plethora of other imaging techniques, technologies, and biomedical research have given us increasing levels of insight into not only of what the brain is actually composed, but as to the brain's functionality. Even still, although we [the human race] are capable of sending robots to Mars and controlling them remotely, we have only become more aware of all that we do not know when it comes to the totality of the human brain. Even still, the limited information available to us regarding the brain is vast, and provides huge insights into just how deeply human beings are connected to chi (bioelectric magnetic energy) and the [individual] psi capabilities many of us involved with chi gung have come to believe and know.

Weighing in slightly over 3 pounds (1.4 kilograms), the human brain is by far the complex and amazing biological product to date. As previously mentioned, it is the controlling agent of the human body's nervous system. The brain itself is comprised of one hundred billion nerve cells; these cells are what people refer to when speaking of "grey matter".

http://www.newscientist.com/article/dn9969-instant-expert-the-human-brain.html?full=true

Along with the "grey", the human brain is also comprised of "white" matter and glial cells. Whereas the grey matter is the neurons, the white matter is the network of axions that connect cells to neurons; these are the axons and dendrites. The glial cells, which represent the ruling majority of the cells in the brain, outnumbering the neurons by ten to one (10:1), amplify neural signals.

The human brain is viewed not only as one structure, but also as having (an): upper brain; lower brain; left and right hemispheres; as well as a many other components, each with specific tasks which they perform.

The "lower" brain, which consists of the spinal cord, brain stem and diencephalons, also contains the following components:

- The medulla regulates blood pressure and breathing and regulating information from the sensory organs;
- The pons relay information regarding movement and spatial awareness which is conveyed from the cerebellum to the [cerebral] cortex;

- The thalamus participates in motor-information exchange
- The hypothalamus controls the hormonal secretions of the pituitary gland and regulates our circadian rythms.

http://health.howstuffworks.com/brain.htm/printable

The "mid brain", represents an area where the higher and lower brains share functionality. Portions of the limbic system rest in both areas, for example; the hypothalamus is more closely aligned with the "lower" brain whereas the amygdala is associated with the "higher" brain.

The limbic system is important in emotional behavior and controlling movements of visceral muscles (see the "Emotional Content" article on the Chi Power blog http://chipower.com/blog/?p=97 for more information regarding the limbic system).

The "higher" brain, which houses the cerebrum, consists of the following components:

- The parietal lobe receives and processes all somatosensory input from the body (touch, pain);
- The frontal lobe is involved in motor skills (including speech) and cognitive functions;
- The occipital lobe receives and processes visual information directly from the eyes and relates this information to the parietal lobe; one of the things it must do is interpret the upside-down images of the world that are projected onto the retina by the lens of the eye;
- The temporal lobe processes auditory information from the ears and relates it to the parietal lobe and the motor cortex of the frontal lobe;
- The insula influences automatic functions of the brainstem and processes taste information;
- The basal ganglia work with the cerebellum to coordinate fine motions, such as fingertip movements

http://health.howstuffworks.com/brain.htm/printable

The cerebrum is the largest part of the human brain and is divided into the left and right hemispheres. Although the interactions between and functionality of each is complex beyond the scope of this article, it is largely viewed that: the right hemisphere is more creative and emotional, specializing in spatial and body awareness, whereas; the left hemisphere deals with logic, speech and language.

http://www.newscientist.com/article/dn9969-instant-expert-the-human-brain.html?full=true

The concept of "consciousness" and where it resides within the brain is widely debated and under intense scrutiny from across the entire scientific community. Biologists, physicists, medical doctors and chemists all play a role in the investigation of where human consciousness resides. Recently, it has been proposed that human consciousness is a result of the direct connection we have with the actual quantum particles via the microtubules within the brain. The interaction of microtubules and quantum energy and the correlations said energy has with chi is something that did not go unnoticed.

In particular, Stuart Hameroff MD has done extensive research and written many papers concerning this and similar topics in relation to the brain, its microtubules, and the inherent quantum behaviors therein.

In his paper, "Chi: A Neural Hologram", Dr. Hameroff details the discovery of the microtubule and its quantum behaviors. Interestingly enough, the specific pathways of the microtubules and their functionality, he notes, correspond strikingly similar to that which Chinese mystics refer to as chi.

"[neural] Microtubules (MT) are hollow cylinders… which are capable of intercepting energy in the far ultra-violet (UV) range… and the upper limit of the narrow window of solar and celestial nonionizing radiation," writes Hameroff.
http://www.quantumconsciousness.org/documents/chi_hameroff_000.pdf

In the program "Supernatural Science: Extra Sensory Perception (Discovery Channel 1999), Hameroff states: "These microtubules are ideally designed quantum computers which makes the connection from our macroscopic world to the microscopic fundamental quantum worlds so we can access and select and taste and experience."

Via neuroimaging techniques, Hameroff was able to observe microtubules flickering "on and off" in a fashion very similar to that of photons and other subatomic particles of the quantum spectrum.

It is the very fact that "subtle magnetic fields have been detected outside the human head… and neuronal generated magnetic fields" which allow neuroimaging to exist."
http://www.quantumconsciousness.org/documents/chi_hameroff_000.pdf

These same fields, this electromagnetic phenomena, is that which we call chi: from the nerve fibers that carry electrical signals throughout the body to the brain's distinct magnetic field to the ion exchange at the cellular level, human beings directly interact with and through electromagnetic energy.

Electricity & Chi: One and the Same

Electricity, defined by Merriam-Webster, is as follows: a fundamental form of energy observable in positive and negative forms that occurs naturally (as in lightning) or is produced (as in a generator) and that is expensed in terms of the movement and interaction of electrons.

Generally speaking, when thinking of electricity, we think of it as something external to our human bodies: the naturally occurring lightning and human created technology being two said instances. There is, however, a form of electricity that is prevalent in every living creature: bioelectricity.

Bioelectricity

Bioelectricity is the electric phenomena related to living organisms.

It is bioelectricity that enables a shark to map the ocean floor. It is bio-electromagnetic phenomena that enable migratory birds to travel great distances at the same time each year with the accuracy we have only been able to reproduce with maps and GPS. It is bioelectricity that enables the electric eel to generate large fields of current outside their bodies.

The difference of electricity vs. bioelectricity is in degree, not in kind. Whereas a lightning bolt can exceed temperatures of 54,000 degrees Fahrenheit (30,000 degrees Celsius), that same current runs through the human body, just on a smaller scale.

In fact, the human body runs largely off of [bio] electricity and has organs dedicated to sensing electromagnetic impulses, both inside and outside the human body. The pineal and pituitary glands are both directly tied to the human body's ability to sense and actively experience electromagnetic phenomenon.

Bioelectricity and the Body

The pineal gland is the evolutionary descendant of our ancestors' ability to perceive light. It also "regulates the circadian rhythms of the body, biological rhythms that are attuned to the day-night cycle," (Celtoslavica, "Electricity and Human Consciousness); these "rhythms" can be and have been disrupted by electromagnetic fields, both naturally occurring as well as man-made. The pituitary gland "controls and influences all other hormonal organs which report back to the pituitary gland" (Celtoslavica, "Electricity and Human Consciousness); in fact, the pituitary gland is largely responsible for the overall functioning and efficiency of the human nervous system. The nervous system in human beings is based entirely off of the ability to transmit electric pulses. Every cell within the human body pumps ions (e.g. that which makes up the quantum field), in and out of the cell for energy purposes; this is called the Sodium-Potassium pump, and can be found in all animal life. Said energy, in the biological animal, is called "adenosine triphosphate" (ATP); biologists and biochemist alike have noted that ATP can be neutral, or carry a charge (plus or minus), and is, infact, a charged particle which the cells use for energy. ATP is the final product of the digestive cycle and further exemplifies the human being's connection (and ability) to experience and manipulate the electromagnetic fields that permeate the Universe. "Bio-magnetism: An Awesome Force in Our Lives", an article published by Reader's Digest (January 1983), highlights some of the [still] cutting edge concepts the scientific community is, and has been, practicing:

> "When a patient with a broken leg that is not healing properly comes to Dr. Basset (Columbia Presbyterian Medical Center in New York City, NY), he is likely to go home with two heavy pads connected by wires to a box that can plug into an electrical wall socket. The patient puts one pad on each side of his broken bone and turns on the device. Coils of wire in the pad induce a pulsing electromagnetic field into his flesh and bone -- a field of energy that somehow commands the bone to heal itself."

As postulated by the scientists interviewed in the article, it makes sense that human beings have the innate ability to sense electromagnetic phenomena:

> "We live on a sun-lit planet, and most living things have acquired some means to use the light. We live in a world filled with sounds, and most living things have developed a means to sense vibrations. Since our planet is also a giant magnet, it should not surprise us to discover that we and many other living things have a sensitivity to Earth's magnetic-force field."

As we look from large-scale physics, e.g., the lightning bolt and the sodium-potassium pump, to smaller scale electromagnetic phenomenon, we find ourselves in the realm of quantum mechanics. Light is an electromagnetic phenomenon. Light is both a wave and a particle. In terms of quantum mechanics, electricity and light are the same. The oscillations of the impulses create the divergent effects. Microwaves, radio waves, even the non-lethal weapons of the US Army (such as the Active Denial System https://www.jnlwp.com/ads.asp) are based out of electromagnetic fields.

Chi and the Body Continued

Chi, too, is an electromagnetic phenomenon. Chi is energy; light energy; bio-electromagnetic energy; electricity. The degree of strength in an electromagnetic impulse is the difference between the heart pumping vs. a heart attack. When building chi, it is important to understand, important to know, that the electricity you are both introducing to your body as well as augmenting within your body, can be controlled/manipulated by your mind; without direct and focused intent, the electrical impulses will be raw, hot, and uncomfortable.

In the previously quoted Reader's Digest article, researchers as far back as 1983 were able to accelerate cellular regeneration in adult rats by intruding electromagnetic waves to afflicted parts of their bodies; humans too, have been shown to have enhanced healing at the cellular level when electromagnet fields are introduced. At the same time, it has been well documented that people exposed to high intensity electromagnetic fields, such as those created by power-line generators, are more susceptible to cancerous develops, such as leukemia.

SPC USA certified instructors teach the Chi Power practitioner how to harness this energy in a healing fashion, without painful side effects. The difference being similar to an invigorating spa- massage vs. being seated in an electric chair at half-power.

Chi, the Inner Circle, and You!

Although the preceding text can be viewed as an article on the Chi Power Blog (http://chipower.com/blog/) it is here in the **Inner Circle** that the depth of such information is explored and cultivated in such a way that it is no longer the high-level scientific theory, but the concrete, life changing reality that comes only with hands-on training and interpersonal instruction.

Chapter 2: The SPC Method

Mental Preparation

One of the very first lessons members of the Inner Circle are taught is the importance of engaging the **mind** with regards to their Chi Power Training. Many scientific studies validate that, with proper mental preparation and active, mindful engagement; you can increase the results of your efforts dramatically.

The importance of engaging the mind is not something that is glossed over; throughout the instructions given, as well as the various articles written by and interviews with Certified Instructors, members of the Inner Circle will read scientific reports validating such claims as well as the pitfalls one can encounter when not being mindful.

Ascending Euphoria

Merriam-Webster defines "euphoria" as follows: "a feeling of well-being or elation". From the very 1st communiqué from Master Instructors Sifu Jones and Sifu Perhacs, members of the Inner Circle are *encouraged* to develop and maintain a euphoric state. In the 9th month, Sifu Perhacs provides a candid video in which he instructs members of the Inner Circle on how to develop and maintain a euphoric state:

- "How you act determines how you feel; not the other way around."
- Read good books that feed your MIND! The habit of beginning at least 5 minutes a day will change your life. Religious doctrines- such as the Bible, help you develop an intimate closeness with the spirit and further enhance your sense of "well-being".
- The laying meditation is something to be enjoyed and sought after: relaxing the physical body is the initial step; after which, or during the process, begin thinking about that which makes you happy and smile.
- Use your affirmations; engage your mind with your affirmations.

The concept of euphoria transcends a simple feeling. The *emotional content* of thought produces energies, which have an impact on your physical reality in many mindboggling ways: from your physical health and psychological to the ability to generate wealth and attract that which you want and desire; the ability to enter and remain in a state of deliberate euphoria defines you as a true "controller".

Affirmations and Autosuggestion

Affirmations and Autosuggestions are two very significant ways to engage the mind and are two major components that set the Chi Power system apart from tradition chi gung methods. Master Instructors Sifu Jones and Sifu Perhacs provide specific instructions with regards to *supercharging* your autosuggestions and affirmations so as to get maximum results regardless of your goals.

Be it increased chi; weight loss; financial success; romantic fulfillment; Master Instructors Sifu Jones and Sifu Perhacs provide the blueprints from which you can tailor to fit your own needs and desires, while gaining unheard of results from the words of your mouth, and thoughts in your mind.

Chi Distillation

When electricity passes through anything, even the human body, some of it is lost and appears in another form of energy: heat. *Chi Distillation* is a technique wherein members of the Inner Circle are given instruction on how to actually cool the energy, cool the body's response to the electricity, and retain the energy without the actual buildup of heat.

By immersing your hands and arms into something cold prior to and while doing your Chi Power exercises, you are making a physical and mental correlation to the nature of the energy being cultivated. As opposed to the traditionally yang chi, which is hot and repelling, members of the Inner Circle engage their minds in such a way that the energy, the chi itself, is both cool and pleasant.

Hot chi is what actually leads to the energy spikes and organ pain as discussed by the Certified Instructors in their Interviews. By keeping the chi cool, the physical body can better enjoy it and respond favorably to the build-up. *Chi Distillation* is one of the very critical aspects to the Chi Power System, allowing members of the Inner Circle to make the types of chi-related gains in a matter of months, which would take other systems a matter of years to achieve.

Physical Exercises

Chi Power is truly a holistic way of developing chi energy. The Body, Mind, and Spirit are engaged in ways so as to: draw a distinction between the three; cultivate a level of sensitivity so as to better identify and enhance the interaction thereof; and promote chi awareness by synergism between the three entities that comprise the Individual.

Bloodwashing

The bloodwashing exercise is the cornerstone of the Chi Power method. This physical exercise directly aids in the development of the body's nerve fibers-which are responsible for the body's ability to harness and circulate the bio-electromagnetic energy referred to in the martial and psi community as "chi".

The bloodwashing exercise ads yet another dimension to chi development. While not only promoting the growth of nerve fibers, which allows the body to carry higher and higher charges of chi, the exercise itself creates a flow-patter that directs the chi in such a way that it actually mimics the rotation and spin of the quantum particles which we are building.

Standing Meditation

The standing meditation is a traditional *yang* exercise that can be done using the cool, euphoric energy that separates the SPC USA Chi Power System from others. The Standing Meditation not only assists the physical body in adjusting to the increasing pressure of the bio-electromagnetic energy, but it also provides an opportunity for the practitioner to engage and "balance" the energy levels in his/her organs.

This exercise, when done properly, can help members of the Inner Circle avoid [unnecessary] painful energy spikes. For those who have been fortunate enough to avoid said symptom, an unpleasant throbbing in the kidneys is just the beginning…

Performed in conjunction with the Bloodwashing and Lying Down meditations, the Standing exercise most certainly prepares the body for advanced levels of extreme chi gung [hence Chi Power] abilities.

Lying Down Meditation

The Lying Down meditation compliments the bloodwashing in the same way that the yin balances the yang in the Taijitu. The Lying Down meditation is the secret to Chi Power, as it teaches the body, mind, and spirit to relax; it is only by relaxing can one truly exercise control over his/her energy.

Oddly enough, the Lying Down meditation is one of the more difficult exercises to master. The act of Lying Down completely still for a set period of time focusing your thoughts on that which is specific (see section on "Autosuggestions and Affirmations") is more challenging than one would think, however; over time, you will learn to use this as an opportunity to truly augment the euphoric feeling and project said energies wherever and to whomever you wish.

Micro/Macro Cosmic Orbits [month 3]

Master Instructors Sifu Jones and Sifu Perhacs dedicate a 45 minute conference call through which members of the Inner Circle can find very detailed information regarding the pros and cons of both the Micro and Macro Cosmic Orbits.

Sifu Jones provides in-depth analysis, sharing with members of the Inner Circle how each orbit affects us both physically as well as psychologically. Although the initial aspects may be positive, generally speaking, continued practice of either exercise over a prolonged period of time will usher bad side effects: dizziness; vertigo; headaches; hormonal imbalances; increased pressure on the pineal and pituitary glands; uneven pressure throughout the body (and its organs).

At any given point, Sifu Jones provides firsthand experiences from himself and [current/previous] students the challenges that face when performing these exercises over a prolonged period of time. Sifu Perhacs also shares with the Inner Circle how he went so far as to develop a hernia from performing the Micro Cosmic Orbit with too much intensity for too long of a period of time.

It is highly recommended that the student follow the instructions given. Regardless of your previous styles or the books you have read, the Chi Power System is a system unlike any other. It would behoove members of the Inner Circle to follow along with the instructions as lain before them so as to maximize their growth and avoid the painful pitfalls that await those that follow the *yang* route.

Chapter 3: The Inner Circle

Welcome

On behalf of Sifu Jones, Sifu Perhacs, the Certified Instructors, and current members within: Welcome to the Inner Circle!

You have taken your first step into a bigger, and brighter world where you will learn not only how to cultivate your energy, but more importantly, how to use your energy for day-to-day success in all of your endeavors. The climb is steep, and the terrain is formidable, however; we can assure you with the dedication of the Master and Certified Instructors and diligence of the Community, we will all reach the Summit of our individual capabilities and goals.

About the IC

The *Inner Circle* is an online community where men and women interested in cultivating and growing their knowledge, awareness, and understanding of *chi* can receive detailed instructions from Masters who have gone before them. Students receive consultation and training techniques/exercises specifically tailored to their level of progression.

Conference calls between the Master Instructors and interviews with Certified Instructor who have trained with the Masters, along with accompanying articles, are available for review via the Inner Circle website. There, members of the Inner Circle have access to a wealth of knowledge, gleaned from the past successes and pitfalls of those who have gone before them.

The Inner Circle is an outlet, which allows members of the Chi Community an opportunity to share experiences. Here, you can join a conversation and add your thoughts, viewpoints, etceteras to assist in not only the growth of others, but yourself as well.

The Nature of Chi

Scientific Premium Company USA takes a holistic approach to Chi Power and the curriculum for the Inner Circle. The thorough nature of the manner in which "chi" is approached provides each student with a complete scientific understanding of chi as well as a practical, utilitarian vantage from day to application and growth.

Circular Chi vs. Linear Chi

Many martial art and chi gung systems promote a *linear* method regarding chi development. Initially, here at SPC USA, students receive instruction in a linear fashion of chi development because this allows students to feel, with certainty, the existence of chi energy and know that they are creators thereof. Knowing that chi is real is one of the most critical steps in Chi Power; this is the crux of the Chi Power Volume 1 instruction.

Although the linear fashions of chi gung provide a much faster buildup, they are limited with regards to their progression. Due to the heavy reliance on hormonal interactions, the abilities of students in linear systems tend to not only plateau, they also endure physical pain directly induced from the unusually hot energy circulating in their bodies which also encourage an inordinate amount of [not always ideal] hormones coursing through the blood stream.

Chi Power Volume 2 begins the transition from linear to circular methods of chi development. Whereas the linear systems focus on hormonal/chemical building which is synonymous with sexual energy, the circular methods directly tie into the electromagnetic aspects of the Universe and engage the spirit. The clockwise flow patterns of the blood washing exercise (BWE) and rotation of the circle exercises match the rotations of the building blocks of the Universe: the subatomic particles of the quantum field.

The difference between the methods is stark. For example, with regards to linear chi, your energy projection is that of radar emissions; energy bounces off of the intended target, and returns back to the sender, including various aspects of the target's energy as well. This means to say, whatever vibrational aspects of the target [please see references on string theory within this document] return to the sender, both good and bad. The circular method provides the chi power practitioner the opportunity to actually *filter* the energy, enabling the adept to decide upon that which they would like to receive into their individual experiences.

Unbeknownst to many involved in chi gung, one of the largest discriminators between those who are able to perform extreme abilities, such as levitate and move objects without physically touching them, is the speed related attribute they are able to attach to their energy. The speeds, which can be achieved, via the circular method are exponentially greater than that of the linear method, and require less effort and are much easier on the physical body and the mind. Tornados are nature's perfect exemplars of the speed of circles; the "eye of the storm" in relation to hurricanes is the calm the Chi Power practitioner represents when performing an extreme technique. The science of centrifugal/centripetal forces show the power achieved through circular rotations. Linear systems simply do not compare.

Three Stages of Chi

Here at SPC USA, we understand that many of the concepts and chi-related experiences that Inner Circle students will be/are experiencing as they begin and continue their Chi Power training are completely foreign and unknown to them. As the practitioner develops his/her chi and sensitivity, general capabilities and awareness make for easily identifiable stages in progression. This is an opportunity for you to be aware of the stages of chi development, so as to not only have a roadmap regarding your own development, but to also provide you with a preview as to what you will experience and what to expect as you move up and through the various stages: Solid; Water and; Gas.

Solid: The *solid* stage of chi is, for many, their initial encounter with chi. This is where neophytes begin to get comfortable with the concept of the energy as well as the feel of the energy. During the *solid* stage, the student focuses on developing emotional stability and awareness via chi distillation; the ability to relax into the energy and enter a state of euphoria is essential to safely progress to and navigate the upper echelon of chi capabilities. It is also during the *solid* stage that students realize the weirdness that

http://www.ChiPowerInnerCircle.com

comes with Chi Power training is the "norm". The *solid* stage is where the foundation is laid.

Water: The *water* stage is both deep and wide. Here, within the *water* stage, Chi Power practitioners experience increased sensitivity to chi energy and begin executing techniques with deliberate and consistent results. The ability to enter a state of euphoria is taken to the next level; here within the *water* stage, the student is able to extend his/her energy and intention and cause others to feel euphoric as well. During the *water* stage, the ability to control the temperature of the chi, as well as individual persons, is consistent and becomes less and less taxing as the student's focus and sensitivity rise. Of great importance during the *water* stage are the gradual openings of the seven vortexes within the body: one in each leg (shin); one in each arm (forearm); one in the torso (belly button); two in the head. As these vortexes open, the Chi Power practitioner becomes aware of vibrations and increased feelings of energy rotations.

Gas: The *gas* stage is the acme of chi development. Here, within the *gas* stage, the Chi Power practitioner is at the apex of his/her abilities, and is truly within the realm of that which is extreme, and able to perform techniques that challenge preconceived notions of the nature of reality. **Please be forewarned:** the *gas* stage is somewhat dangerous in nature. The amount of energy coursing through the body is at a level which is almost unbearable and is difficult on the mind, as time-space morphs in ways that are not easily expressed via language nor the written word; hence the need to master the technique of chi distillation and euphoria early in your progression).

Light Chi & Heavy Chi

Not only are there different "stages" of chi, there are different properties of chi as well. The major dichotomy of chi resides in the realm of *light* or *heavy* chi.

Light chi is both light in color as well as light in weight. *Light* chi has an "airy" quality. As a building block of *heavy* chi (discussed below), it is within the arena of *light* chi that the desired attributes of your chi are programmed. Generally, this means that over time and with practice, your chi naturally takes on the sensations of "cool" and "euphoric". *Light* chi directly affects the emotions and should be cultivated in a way that is conducive to well-being.

Heavy chi is thick, and malleable. There is an increased particle density in regards to *heavy* chi, which allows for and leads to "formed" chi[3]. The general attributes of *heavy* chi are hot, naturally destructive, and somewhat unmanageable; although it is relatively easy to form, it is a challenge to hold the specific shape and keep the energy cool. In fact, for this reason, heavy chi instruction begins within the Closed Door system, as the margin for error significantly decreases

---

[3] "Formed" chi is chi that takes on specific shapes and properties to be used for advanced techniques; formed chi is taught in the Closed Door System, as it is somewhat dangerous if not done correctly.

http://www.ChiPowerInnerCircle.com

Nutrition and Chi Power

Dr. Thomas Earnest, a member of the IC, was kind enough to share his expertise with the Inner Circle during an information session with Master Sifus Jones and Perhacs. Dr. Earnest is a practicing clinical nutritionist with a background in Oriental Medicine.

Dr. Earnest went into great detail, listing the pros and cons of every major food group, providing the Inner Circle with best practices regarding nutrition and eating habits as well as debunking myths around food and nutrition. Of great value are the notes he provided that can be found in the month 12 curriculum in the form of a .pdf. Here, he provides resources for additional information and verification of that which he shared during the information session.

Nutrition should be of great concern for those of us practicing chi power. According to Dr. Earnest, "the better [health of] the body the easier it is to get chi out and build." The alarming situation for many of us is that we are **overfed** and *under nourished*. With great detail, accuracy, and passion, Dr. Earnest shares with us an eating and nutrition plan which provides a transformation at every level.

For example, Dr. Earnest assures us that the old maxim of "you get what you pay for" is unfortunately true, especially when it comes to food and nutritional supplements. Our mindset as a culture, willing to pay top dollar for luxury items fails us when we go "bargain hunting" at the grocery stores; food is that which we use to fuel our lives. A high quality, nutrition-filled diet provides us with energy and health benefits so many of us are lacking and searching. Fortunately, Dr. Earnest lays out an eating plan for the IC showing us how to reclaim our health. From notions of macrobiotics to good fats, weight loss strategies, the wonders of coconut oil to how best to eat vegetables for maximum vitamin intake, Dr. Earnest gives the Inner Circle priceless nuggets of information on how to eat our ways to a better quality of life. Make sure you have a pen and paper handy when listening to this information session.

Chapter 4: Inner Circle Curriculum

Techniques and Building Blocks

First and foremost: chi is not magic. The extreme, fantastic abilities of martial arts masters of old are real. They are techniques that were honed over the years by men and women who were very dedicated and mindful to their training.

The speed at which you develop your abilities and hone the techniques is entirely up to you. By following the path lain by Master Instructors Sifu Jones and Sifu Perhacs, you will see that Chi Power affects everything and every aspect of your life, from: financial success; interpersonal relationships [romantic and otherwise]; physical health and mental well being. Chi Power is not just for martial artists; although the physical techniques of increased speed and awareness lend themselves easily to the martial domain, Chi Power can be applied in everyday situations.

Again, the techniques taught within the curriculum, highlighted in the sections to follow, give you an overview of the natural progression of abilities as well as the how's and why's each exercise is important, and how mastering said technique prepares the student for the extreme, psi related abilities for which they yearn to cultivate.

Telekinesis and Psi abilities

Telepathy, clairvoyance, telekinesis and other "psi" related abilities are often the end goals of many who seek to cultivate and harness their chi: the ability to "know" or "sense" the thoughts and intentions of others; the ability to see from a distance, without physically being there; the ability to move objects; levitation; these are the things members of the Inner Circle are preparing themselves for as they better harness their chi and better attune their minds, bodies, and spirits.

These abilities are in and of themselves *extreme*, and it takes a great deal of time, concentrated effort, and commitment to activate and achieve these abilities. As previously noted by the sections covering the scientific aspect of chi, none of this is magic. These are techniques that you learn over a period of time, and master with diligent practice. Members of the Inner Circle are privy to audio and video files of our Certified Instructors demonstrating [some] of these abilities to help encourage you to reach higher and further- to know that you too can go beyond the boundaries imposed by the ordinary.

Using Chi to Bend Metal

Certified Instructor, Sifu Andrei Biesinger demonstrates one of the ways in which he uses chi in his everyday life. As a mechanic, Sifu Andrei Biesinger is often faced with the challenge of bending pipes and metal objects that require an unusual amount of physical exertion and unwieldy tools.

"Using Chi to Bend Metal": http://chipower.com/blog/?p=70

Andrei developed a technique where he pulses his chi through the metal, and softens it, so he can bend the objects with minimum to no effort. Not only can the video be seen on the Chi Power Training blog, but also, members of the Inner Circle are also privy to candid conversations between Certified Instructor Sifu Andrei Biesinger and Master Instructors Sifu Jones and Sifu Perhacs.

Got Skills?

Sifu Perhacs introduced a video series where members of the Inner Circle demonstrate some of their external [chi] manipulation abilities. While the individuals themselves remain anonymous, the footage is real and the techniques shown unadulterated.

The goal of these videos is simple: the Inner Circle is a Community of Practice, where men and women desiring to learn, explore, and grow their chi abilities can commune and share experiences and techniques. In short, the videos showcased encourage every member, from the 1st day beginning to the Certified Instructor Level, to increase our enthusiasm and exuberance.

For example, psi-like abilities, such as *telekinesis* are demonstrated in multiple ways. In one such video, a member of the Inner Circle shows the ability to move a piece of folded paper within the confines of a closed compact disc case. In a similar video, a member of the Inner Circle places a ping-pong ball inside the clear plastic housing of a compact disc spindle and causes the ping-pong ball to move in a circular pattern.

Again, the goal of these videos is to demonstrate what is possible when the chi practitioner opens his/her mind to the possibilities, and [most importantly] follows the instructions set forth by Master Instructors Sifu Jones and Sifu Perhacs. The Inner Circle is truly a Community or Practice: as the old adage goes- "Iron sharpens Iron".

Sensing Objects

In a video for the members of the Inner Circle, Certified Instructor Andrei Biesinger is challenged by Master Instructor Sifu Perhacs to demonstrate his level of chi sensitivity by identifying objects.

The video of the demonstration is amazing in and of itself. The techniques are simple to master through practice, and are the building blocks for future abilities upon which growth and augmentation can be achieved.

Sensing Colors

Early in the training curriculum for the Inner Circle, Master Instructors Sifu Jones and Sifu Perhacs introduce the concept of sensing colors with chi energy. The exercises are deceptively simple, and the technique rather easy to master. It is taught early in the training, as this is a cornerstone of "sensitivity" training, and leads to the ability to somatically sense things not readily seen with the physical eye (you do this exercise with eyes closed or blind-folded) or verbally spoken.

Scientifically speaking, colors are associated with different wavelengths of light; each wavelength has a specific energy and this energy is expressed in both color and *heat*. The initial ability to sense the nuances between shades and contrasts of colors is what leads to the ability to actually manipulate and change objects, very similar to alchemy. In his book, The Elegant Universe, Pulitzer Prize Finalist Dr. Brian Greene shares with the scientific community: "For electromagnetic waves in the visible part of the spectrum, an increase in frequency corresponds to a change in color from red to orange to yellow to green to blue to indigo and finally to violet. For some unknown reason, the color of the impinging light beam – not its total energy – controls whether or not electrons are ejected, and if they are, the energy they have."

Furthermore: "each successive element has a lower ionization energy because it is easier to remove an electron since the atoms are less tightly bound."

Linking one scientific truth to the other, a logician's "if/then" began:

- if chi is bio-electromagnetic energy

- and electromagnetic energy and light are one and the same

- and the color of the light wave (frequency) is what ejects electrons

- and the difference between elements are based solely upon their number of electrons

Then: the ability to sense colors, and one-day change the color of a light wave ultimately leads to alchemy.

Merrian-Webster defines alchemy as follows:

1 : a medieval chemical science and speculative philosophy aiming to achieve the transmutation of the base metals into gold, the discovery of a universal cure for disease, and the discovery of a means of indefinitely prolonging life

2 : a power or process of transforming something common into something special

3 : an inexplicable or mysterious transmuting

The difference between the elements in the Periodic Table of Elements is solely based around said element's electron composition; add one or remove one, and you have a completely different element. For example, Hydrogen (H) has 1 orbiting electron; Helium (He) has 2 orbiting electrons. Lead (Pb), which has 82 orbiting electrons, can be transmuted to gold (Au) upon removing 3 electrons.

Mastering color sensing, and thereafter, changing the actual color of the visible light, places alchemy within our grasps. The amount of energy, and the ability to control said energy, is what differentiates neophytes from experts; being able to manipulate the structure of the chemical composition of an object can not only come in handy (read Paulo Coelho's The Alchemist), but lead to a level of sensitivity and control that will act as the springboard to even greater abilities.

OBE

The Out of Body Experience is a technique members of the Inner Circle are taught so as to better get in touch with their spirits. The OBE is a *yin* technique that although many have experienced by accident, through practicing relaxation techniques, members of the Inner Circle will learn to perform the OBE at will.

The Out of Body Experience is technique that is very similar to the psi-related ability remote viewing. Learning to release and direct the spirit with the mind is a technique that takes effort, however; once mastered, it can provide the adept with a source of uncanny information.

Remote Viewing & Astral Projection

With the assistance of a certified instructor, Sifu Perhacs shares with the Inner Circle the initial steps in performing the psi technique of "remote viewing".

http://www.ChiPowerInnerCircle.com

Remote viewing is akin to sending a feeling out at first, which comes back to like a picture in the mind. Astral projection is similar to sending a part of the spirit into the area in question; this technique provides a richer and more detailed amount of information and situational awareness when compared to remote viewing, however; astral projection is more difficult in nature as it requires sensitivity to and awareness of the spirit. The easiest way to begin astral projection is via remote viewing. After a period of time and practice, the increased sensitivity of remote viewing gradually changes over to astral projection: a complete metamorphosis takes place when you are able to feel and use your spirit. Astral projection takes a little bit of the spirit to the place you want to go; Out of Body Experiences (OBEs) take the whole spirit-body to where you want to go.

The video provides systematic instructions to assist in the development of these techniques, with the initial step of learning to feel other people inside another room. Although using a partner is ideal, especially having one who can project chi energy for initial ease of sensitivity and awareness, Sifu Perhacs provides a .pdf document that highlights different ways of performing this technique, one of which can be done alone. One of most important aspects of performing this technique is the need to be relaxed; the deeper you can relax and enter a "yin state", the better your sensitivity and results will be.

Advanced Healing Techniques

Of great interest to many in the Inner Circle are healing techniques. In this video, Sifu Perhacs demonstrates the best practices and methods when using energy to heal.

Sifu Perhacs takes time to debunk popular misconceptions centered on healing with energy, and goes several steps further; Sifu Perhacs divulges SPC USA Chi Power trade secrets as he demonstrates healing techniques with the assistance of certified instructor Sifu Brown. During the demonstration, Sifu Perhacs engages cool chi in conjunction with soft tones and quasi-hypnotic suggestions to relax his patient. As the demonstration ends, it is clear by Sifu Brown's responses that he was in a trance and that the techniques performed by Sifu Perhacs revitalized him as though waking from a "power nap".

As with many of the information videos, instructions highlighting the process as well as non-obvious tips are provided as a .pdf document.

Transferring Energy: Hot and Cold Temperatures

Sifu Andrei Biesinger demonstrates his impressive skills yet again in this Inner Circle video exclusive. The concept of chi distillation is based upon the mind's ability to control/manipulate the temperature of energy. Sifu Biesinger takes this concept and shows a real-world application of not only cooling down the chi, but actually transferring heat energy from one object to another; all documented via his laser guided thermometer and video camera.

The individual applications are endless for each practitioner. For healers, the ability to lower the temperature of the inflamed area *without* absorbing said negative energy into you is ideal. The ability to simply cool off and remain physically cool so as to avoid overheating and the accompanying unflattering perspiration during, let's say, public/professional gatherings (see section on Pheromones) goes a long way. The ability to generate heat when cold and/or influence the temperature of a person or object in general can be of significant value when the tactic is properly married with the strategy of win-win.

This skill warrants further investigation and competency on the part of each member of the Inner Circle.

The Law of Attraction

Sifu Jones and Sifu Perhacs hosted a very special conference regarding "The Law of Attraction" (as made famous by The Secret) for members of the Inner Circle. It is a very powerful seminar, filled with information and actual techniques people can use in conjunction with their chi to not only attract what they want, but more importantly: how to do it and get the results they want with greater and greater specificity.

Members of the Inner Circle know that the mind is a key factor in developing one's chi. This is important, as what we are sharing has been verified throughout the scientific community and "taken for granted" by the general populace, but not investigated to the same level as what the Certified Instructors implement in our daily lives.

In his book Entangled Minds, Dean Radin discusses the "Double slit experiment" where photons (light particles) are observed to determine if light is either a particle or a wave. Without going into the technical details, it has been determined that light is both a particle and a wave at the same time. [For those interested in the specifics of the experiment, please see pages 211-212 of Entangled Minds]. Here is where it gets interesting: it is what the observer expects the particle's behavior to be that actually determines/influences the outcomes of the results. This is not to say that the experiment is fixed; the men and women of the scientific community performing this experiment (over many many years) have done so in the most rigorous and controlled facilities. **No cheating allowed!** However, the results of this experiment have been verified and repeated by physicists around the world: the observer's expectations of the system actual determine the outcome of the experiment. On a microscopic level, where the actual building blocks of the universe take place, we can influence their behavior with our minds and expectations.

Later in Entangled Minds, we find the following:

> "This concept has been studied in hundreds of experiments with teachers, attorneys, judges, business managers, and health care providers. It has been repeatedly shown that expectations unintentionally affect the responses of research participants, pupils, jurors, employees, and parents." (pg 286).

This is to say that we actually influence the outcome of events on a macroscopic, large scale, level as well as at the atomic level.

Pheromones

Merriam-Webster online dictionary defines "pheromone" as follows: a chemical substance that is usually produced by an animal and serves especially as a stimulus to other individuals of the same species for one or more behavioral responses. We draw upon biochemistry and share with members of the Inner Circle community: how chi affects the pheromones and; what we as chi gung practitioners can do to stack the deck in our favor.

Pheromones[4] are picked up by the olfactory senses subconsciously. We are generally unaware of the specific chemical messages an individual sends, however; research has shown that the [pheromone] stimulation of olfactory senses allows the pheromone to "directly influence the neuroendocrinology of emotions" (James V. Kohl et al; Human Pheromones: Integrating Neuroendocrinology and Ethology: Invited Nel Review).

Later in the same article, Kohl and his associates state: "the affect of pheromones on our emotions is linked to the effect of pheromones on the hormones of the hypothalamic-pituitary- gonadal axis –an unconscious affect." Please keep the reference of the "hypothalamic-pituitary- gonadal axis" in mind. SPC made a special note regarding the pituitary gland and its role in bio-electromagnetic phenomena (chi) in the following article: "Qigong, Electricity & The Human Body"; http://chipower.com/blog/?p=47#more-47. The article which provided the specific pituitary reference can be found here: "Electricity and Human Consciousness" by Celtoslavica; http://www.celtoslavica.de/bibliothek/electricity.html.

Pheromones: "Yin and Yang"

The two male pheromones associated with having a physiological and behavioral response in females are androstenol and androstenone. Interesting enough, one of these pheromones attracts partners whereas the other repels. Laboratory experiments have shown "the application of androstenone to females led to negative descriptions of males whereas the application of androstenol led to a description of males as being sexually attractive," (Vohl et al). It would make sense, then, for men to maximize the output of androstenol and minimize the production of androstenone. Unfortunately, like yin-yang, you cannot have one without the other.

Androstenone is a byproduct of the oxidation of androstenol. It is androstenol that the body initially produces however; it is often quickly converted to androstenone via the chemical reaction called oxidation. The challenge, then, is to slow down the oxidation process of androstenol, in an attempt to maximize an individual male's pheromone attractiveness.

Pheromones and Chi

Electricity can come in many forms, be it bio-electromagnetic energy, or various types of specific radiations: electricity is electricity. Electricity also plays a very important role in oxidation: Oxidation describes the loss of electrons by a molecule, atom or ion. At the molecular level, as androstenol looses electrons, it becomes androstenone. In this sequence of events, the male pheromone, initially of the "attracting" sort, turns into that which is "repelling". The similarities between male pheromones and "chi", yin-yang, should be very much apparent at this point. Let us take it one step further.

The act of oxidation, the removal of an electron, is (on a quantum scale), an act of repelling; the electromagnetic phenomenon of "heat" energy plays a role in this chemical reaction of large-scale physics.

Logically speaking, then, if a man were somehow able to control, at a subatomic level,

---

[4] Although the content of this section is available on the Chi power Syndicate blog, members of the Inner Circle have access to an .mp3 recording between Certified Instructor Don Brown, author of said articles, and Master Instructor Sifu Jones; there, Members of the Inner Circle receive additional information not contained within the article at a greater level of detail

the amount of heat his bio-electromagnetic energy produced, he would have an uncanny advantage over other men with regards to his pheromone properties of attraction. He would be able to significantly slow the process of androstenol (attracting pheromone) turning into androstenone (repelling pheromone).

Although this seems somewhat abstract, when applying the concepts of chi generation, especially with regards to the attributes of yin (soft, cool, relaxing energy) versus yang (hot, aggressive, repelling energy), the concepts dovetail nicely. By cultivating cool chi, and focusing on the attributes of cool soft, relaxing energy, the body, on a quantum level, will produce bio-electromagnetic energy that is slow to oxidize the pheromones. In fact, men who cultivate this type of energy not only "attract" like a human magnet, but are often looked upon and viewed as more "attractive", without having done anything of outward significance. These small changes in perception and focus, at a very microscopic level, will in fact, have huge results in the large-scale world of interacting with other people.

Pheromones and the Inner Circle

Members of the Inner Circle receive specific instructions and additional information so as to communicate information provided by the latest scientific data to assist in achieving their individual goals. As the poet John Donne penned hundreds of years ago: "No man is an island". Because we need to interact with others, it is always in our best interest to be attracting that which will assist us; if we can somehow get others to want to help us, at all times, we will have managed to stack the odds in our individual favor. We want you to be successful and we have developed many products and courses to help you maximize your inner potential and bring your very best to the forefront.

Emotional Content

Emotional-content[5] is an enigmatic concept that is difficult to grasp and at the same time, has concrete ramifications in the quality of life for chi gung practitioners.

Chi Power, as taught by Instructors Sifu Jones and Sifu Perhacs embraces the concept of "emotional content", and the specific techniques on how to use it to the practitioners advantage is part of the Inner Circle curriculum.

In this article, we will provide you with some biology-based principles that show exactly what emotions are made of and provide a glimpse as to how this will affect your chi.

According to Merriam-Webster, an emotion is: "a conscious mental reaction (as anger or fear) subjectively experiences as strong feeling usually directed toward a specific object and typically accompanied by physiological and behavioral changes in the body." It is that last portion of the definition on which this article will focus: physiological and behavioral changes in the body.

Hormones: The Building Blocks of Emotions

---

[5] Although the content of this section is available on the Chi power Syndicate blog, members of the Inner Circle have access to an .mp3 recording between Certified Instructor Don Brown, author of said articles, and Master Instructor Sifu Jones; there, Members of the Inner Circle receive additional information not contained within the article at a greater level of detail

According to Dr. Barry Sears, there are only two hormones upon which all emotions are based. "The two primary mediators of emotions are cytokines (hormones that are involved in inflammation) and eicosanoids."
http://www.cbn.com/health/NaturalHealth/drsears_mindbodydiet.aspx
Cytokines and eicosanoids come in multiple flavors; all of which have a specific role to play. It should be noted, however, that some of these hormonal derivatives do, in fact, have an overarching negative impact on the body, especially those which encourage inflammation; these types of inflammatory producing hormones are not only associated with depression (unusually large amounts of such agents have been found in the spinal fluid of suicide victims), but have also been shown to adversely affect the production of natural killer cells in the body as they are the main source of the stress hormone cortisol.

As an aside:

According to Dr. Esther Sternberg of the National Institute of Mental Health: "A chronically stressed brain orders release of hormones and other chemicals that tamp down the immune system so it can't fight off disease or speed healing. Too much stress even ages us faster." http://www.msnbc.msn.com/id/29353787/

It should be noted that the human brain stores and generates "emotions" in its limbic system. The limbic system itself is comprised of connections of glands and structures that are located on top of the brainstem and are buried under the cortex.

"Limbic system structures are involved in many of our emotions and motivations, particularly those that are related to survival. Such emotions include fear, anger, and emotions related to sexual behavior. The limbic system is also involved in feelings of pleasure that are related to our survival, such as those experienced from eating and sex."
http://biology.about.com/od/anatomy/a/aa042205a.htm

There are two members of the limbic system which will serve well to illustrate a very important point that is often stressed to members of the Inner Circle: building chi pressure in and running extreme amounts of chi through the brain is something that is rarely recommended. The sheer amount of electromagnetic pressure along with the stimulation of the receptors of the cells that comprise the limbic system can, in fact, cause the brain to dump large amounts of hormones into the blood stream and throughout the body. The results can often be disastrous, as each gland produces a specific series of cytokines and eicosanoids; not knowing what, which, how and why could easily lead the chi gung practitioner into a hormonal roller coaster ride that is neither fun nor exciting.

The Limbic System's Significant Contributors

The hypothalamus is about the size of a pearl, and directs a multitude of important functions. It regulates the body's circadian rhythms, and is "an important emotional center, controlling the molecules that make you feel exhilarated, angry, or unhappy."
http://biology.about.com/od/anatomy/a/aa042205a.htm
The hypothalamus is responsible for the production of what is called the: Corticotropin-releasing hormone (CRH). Abnormal levels of this specific inflamatory hormone has been found in the cerebrospinal fluid of suicide victims.
The hypothalamus also produces Dopamine, which is believed to provide a teaching signal to parts of the brain responsible for acquiring new behavior, similar to Pavlovian

dogs. It also produces Somatostatin, suppresses the release of pancreatic hormones, thus inhibiting the release of insulin and glucagon.
http://en.wikipedia.org/wiki/Hypothalamus
The amygdala, another significant contributor to the Limbic System, directly affects activities like friendship, love and affection, on the expression of mood and, mainly, on fear, rage and aggression The amygdala is also the center for identification of danger, which is fundamental for self preservation.
http://biology.about.com/library/organs/brain/blamygdala.htm
With those two very simple examples, it should be quite apparent as to why sending energy into the head could potentially create disastrous results. Inadvertently increasing or decreasing the production of Somatostatin, for example, could, in fact, have diabetic ramifications of a period of time; as this is the hormone directly involved in suppressing the release of insulin and glucagons.
Causing the amygdala to function in a hyperactive way could for example, cause an individual to confuse the emotional response of something that is dangerous and life threatening with that which is safe and pleasurable.
Although somewhat innocent and well meaning on the surface, running chi through the head could, in fact, have life threatening (and certainly altering) results.
[Although the preceding information available on the Chi power Syndicate blog, members of the Inner Circle have access to an .mp3 recording between Certified Instructor Don Brown, author of said articles, and Master Instructor Sifu Jones; there, Members of the Inner Circle receive additional information not contained within the article at a greater level of detail to further enhance their "attracting" abilities.]

Chi Training Partner

A training partner when doing Chi Power is someone all of us should have. A training partner can assist our growth and help us stay mindful of energies. A training partner can also help you grow and develop your chi faster. There is, unfortunately, a "catch".
In a conference call hosted between Sifu Jones and Sifu Perhacs, members of the Inner Circle are given the parameters of the characteristic they need to look for and attract when seeking out a chi training partner. The aforementioned pros are certainly worthwhile. The cons, however, can be shockingly unpleasant.
The specific and determined comingling of energies is, in fact, the pinnacle of intimacy. Therefore, the person with whom you decide to engage as a chi training partner should, at bare minimum, be like-minded and of the same gender. Stark differences in religion, morality, spirituality and the like can unfortunately turn your chi partner into [potentially] your worst enemy should the energies comingle and create a *yang* level of destructive interference; and this person will, undoubtedly, *know* you. Similarly, unless your training partner is your husband or wife, this will avoid sexually related pitfalls sure to come.
Although a training partner can be a good barometer and help you grow, Sifu Jones and Sifu Perhacs forewarn members of the Inner Circle the dangers in choosing the wrong partners, as they have done in the past. Like all of the conference calls, the message is clear, candid, and full of the wisdom learned from life experiences. A good chi training partner is a good thing; a bad chi training partner is terrible in ways that cannot be summed-up with words.

Chapter 5: Inner Circle Community

Questions & Answers Sessions and Topics

Every month, at least once a month (sometimes more than) Master Instructors Sifu Jones and Sifu Perhacs provide very detailed responses to various emails that have been collected throughout the month. Often they will use the nature of the questions posed to serve as barometers regarding to the development and challenges of the overarching membership of the Inner Circle.

Below you will find a pertinent list of the questions asked by members of the Inner Circle; the answers to which have been addressed by Master Instructors Sifu Jones and Sifu Perhacs and are available for members of the Inner Circle to review at their leisure via the Inner Circle web portal. The questions come in the form of phone calls, emails, and are answered on a personal, one-on-one level. However, not only are the questions captured for future reference for members of the Inner Circle, but shared (anonymously) so that everyone can benefit from this Community.

Regardless of your level or understanding, within each Question and Answer session, there is something to be gained by everyone.

Q & A Session 1

- Can you practice the blood washing and other exercises outside?

- The books say not to practice in the cold, you say it's okay, which is right? Are there problems with doing exercises in the cold?

- After doing the lying down meditation is it normal to be in a fog for a while afterwards? Sometimes it's hard to get back up, is there a way to stop this side effect?

- Is there anything for people, who can't sleep because they are use to staying up all night?

- Should you put the tongue to the roof of the mouth or tighten up the anus muscles while doing the Vol-1 DVD exercises like when doing the atom exercise?

- Is it usual to feel static electricity while walking thru doorways or to feel peoples' energy bounce off you when they point at you?

- Are there going to be any other type side effects with this?

- Should we still be practicing the Chi Power Plus exercises?

- Are there other exercises that expand the nerve fibers besides the blood washing exercise?

- When doing the cross one leg over the other exercise, I can feel the sensations in one leg, but not so much in the other one. Why?

- I heard you mention yin & yang a bunch of times, what is the difference between the two?

- If I have trouble standing in place is there something else I can do besides the standing meditation?

- How come I feel the energy go down parts of my body, but I can't feel it in others? Will this change with these exercises?

- It seems like I feel the energy more when I don't actually touch my skin then when I do. Is this normal? Is it okay to do it this way? I've been doing chi gung for 10-years and feel the energy fine

- How long does it take to get the chi distillation technique down? My chi seems to be hot all the time, even with the ice, any suggestions?

- Why does your method say to use a cool & good feeling, when other methods are doing the hard breaths & sounds?

Q & A Session 2

- Sometimes when I'm pushing energy thru someone's body, it will come to an area that won't push thru and they would feel a zing of energy, is this normal and how dangerous is it to push the energy on thru?

- I can make the magnetic feeling between my hands when I do the palm test, but I can't seem to move an object. Why won't it move an object, but I feel it okay? How do I get the object to move? Is there a technique to learn that causes you to move the object?

- What does circular chi mean?

- Does it help to do the lying down meditation?

- Will weight training hurt my chi power training?

- Does doing the Blood Washing exercises help with arterial plaque and hardening of the arteries? How about cancers?

- Is it possible to space travel, or do things as warping or distorting space or time? Can you appear in distant places at will?

- Is it dangerous to stimulate parts of the brain that have latent abilities?

- Will my chi accidentally cause damage to computer stuff or sensitive equipment like software?

- How do I speed up the healing process for injuries?

- Is there a correlation between dark matter and chi energy?

- If my chi attracts demons or bad spirits will I have defend myself?

- Should I be avoiding certain foods or chemicals or drugs like aspirin? Will taking them impact my chi?

- Do I need to know about nutrition and how does this affect my chi?

Q & A Session 3

- What is Wu Chi?

- What is circle walking or walking in a figure 8 pattern?

- What is Tai Chi/Chi Kung Ruler?

- Will we be covering the martial aspects of chi kung?

- Will we be going over any of these type techniques in our training?

- After building my chi sometimes when I take a shower I feel somewhat claustrophobic-is this normal or am I yanging too much?

- Does it make a difference whether my door is open or closed in my chi room?

- How am I going to be effected if I am constantly working on people I don't know like in my reiki practice?

- I was doing the energy too hard and the over flow went into my kidneys and now I can't train without pain, what should I do? Is there a way to speed up the time I have to wait so I can train again?

- Should we use the same objects you use in the sensing objects video or can we pick ones of our own?

- I have been trying to sense objects like you showed in the video, but can't get any of them right, do you have any suggestions to make it easier?

- Can a chi master influence or control the outcome of games of chance, sports, casinos, ect.?

- Is densified or condensed chi the same as ectoplasm?

- What's your take on pyramid energy, chi generators and Crystal quartz?

- What's your take on the Tibetan five rights which they say produce a rejuvenating effects?

- The other day while talking with someone, who was describing them self going thru a panic attack, I started having chest pains myself-is this kind of thing normal? Do you think there is something wrong with me, he was having any symptoms just describing them?

- Sometimes I feel pulsations in my ears during meditations and sometimes even without meditating and the pulses don't match my heart rate-is this normal or is there something wrong with my ears?

Q & A Session 4

- What is the main source of chi we are using, is it from the air, food & water?

- Can breathing from the left nostril only cause your body to cool down and breathing from only the right nostril heat you back up? Would this be an effective technique to use in order to cool my chi?

- I like doing the blood washing exercise, but sometimes when I do it for more than an hour, I notice I get a lot of lower back pain, which seems to pulse, is this normal to feel? Is there a way around this pain as I suffer from lower back pain enough?

- Lately, after doing my exercises and I finish with the lying down med, when I get back up I feel a rush of energy taking over my body (it's a good feeling energy-not really cool yet), but it seems to be everywhere, is the chi suppose to feel like this? Is this what you mean by the water stage? What is jing energy and should I be cultivating it?

- You told us about being able to speed up some one's heart and slowing it down-could you explain it further? I'm not sure what I'm supposed to do in order to do that.

- Will the Vol-1 DVD take you to a level where you can see and hear dead people?

- If I only bought the Vol-1 DVD and didn't get any future volumes would I still get good enough to move something like of significance?

- I know you said I might feel sensations in my ears and around my body (like sounds and movements), but lately when I have been doing my exercises, I have been hearing cracking, Crunching, and popping sounds, like electricity sometimes does when it is overloading a line, does this mean I'm overloading myself?

- Sometimes in my lying down meditation I can hear faint voices talking, but I can't figure out what they are saying. Is it normal to pick up voices while practicing this kind of chi gung?

Q & A Session 5

- Can a chi master diagnose illness or disease with accuracy?

- Will chi practice improve my eye sight or hearing ability? How about the other senses?

- What abilities can we expect by the end of the first year or the second year?

- Can the money earned in gambling by using chi power, be cleansed by the chi energy?

- You talk about using chi energy in other applications, could you say use it for getting a better job or even getting one?

- I was trying the pulsing technique on my brother, but he said he couldn't feel anything. Am I doing something wrong? I told myself I wanted him to feel it?

- In the chi power plus material, you show us how to attract animals to us by using the yin chi breath, is that the way we are going to learn how do this in the inner circle? Should I start practicing that kind of breath in order to be ready, when we learn it?

- How long does it take to bend metals (psychokinesis)?

- When I get up from my lying down med, I can easily feel the chi moving around me, is it because I'm just getting more sensitive due to being motionless or do you actually build up your chi during the lying down med too?

- On a similar note, I can wiggle my fingers now and feel the sensations all around my body from doing it, is this because I'm just more sensitive (and there's the same amount of chi) or is it a case that my chi is building up and I'm feeling it more due to the build up?

- You have said that yelling and shouting doesn't mesh well with this method, I'm an instructor and need to shout sometimes, so everyone can hear, will this be a problem? How about using extreme laughter, is it also bad?

- My question is regarding while sleeping, is it dangerous to have your arms/hands lying on your chest? If you were deep breathing while dreaming and your limbs were on your chest would it hurt you? I was doing a lying down med and when I got up a rush of chi energy went shooting down into my leg and foot after I clenched my hand in a fist. In an mp3 you said we don't know where those breaths will go, will I get hurt accidentally doing them in dreams?

- Let's say I had to quit training for a couple weeks, does your nerve fibers still grow for awhile after you stop? How much chi would I be losing?

- I'm having the hardest time putting out the candle, could you give me any suggestions to make it easier?

- Something new happening, I am starting to get shocked a lot just walking across carpeting. Is this because the chi energy is getting stronger and jumping out of me? Is this how we are going to get something to move in the future?

Q & A Session 6

- Since chi is made up of sub atomic particles, is it possible, once you've gotten good enough at it to materialize a solid object? Also I heard of putting up barriers, is it possible to put up an actual physical wall as opposed to an etheric barrier (a mentally perceived barrier) to protect from psychic attacks?

- About how long does it take to get to the water stage? I realize it varies, but what is a typical time range? Also how strong would one's chi abilities be at this point?

- If one exercises, but not on a regular consistent basis, would the chi still build up over a longer period of time?

- Aside from building up the chi thru the exercises, is it necessary to practice projecting the chi all the time in order to get good? Will you still get good not practicing the projecting, but just do the exercises?

- When using auto suggestions to manifest something like a larger income, is it necessary to consciously work at the goal with the chi providing the opportunity, or will the chi just automatically increase the income?

- Speaking of auto suggestions, is it possible to use them in order to speed up the results of your training?

- Besides from the martial arts and health benefits, what are some real time applications for chi?

- I have been doing some heavy work and my muscles were sore, so I pulsed down the chi thru my sore muscles and the pain went away. Is it a good idea to use pulsing techniques to get rid of pain? Also I wear a rosary around my neck, will it get charged up with chi energy? Does anything that touches you or around you get charged up?

- You keep reminding us to make the chi exercises in a happy blissful state, by that do you mean a calm happiness or more of an excited happiness?

- My energy fields have started to expand as far as I can spread my arms apart and I've noticed I feel energy around me in any direction and it feels like when I do the palm test, have you experienced this before?

- To what extent do we create our own reality? Also is shape shifting possible?

- Quick question about bone marrow/energy packing and the blood washing exercise, when we do those exercises are we taking the energy that is around us & using it to increase our psi & energy? Is it actually that simple?

- What should the ratio or balance be for the micro/macro cosmic orbits? I can feel the energy more doing it in the reverse way is this normal?

- I have been using the ice, trying to learn the chi distillation technique, how do you know when you have got it down? My body seems to feel cold all the time now, so much so that I have started to get pains coming out of my joints, is this suppose to feel like this?

- I started practicing trying to put the candle out to see if it would really go out like you guys say it would and I actually was able to put it out after I cut down the wick. I was wondering though if your eyes are suppose to tear up as I found mine kept doing so as I concentrated harder, is this normal & is it safe to do? .

Q & A Session 7

- Why is the BWE done so fast? Is this important (the fast moving part) or can I do the exercise much slower, so it doesn't make me sweat so much?

- So, it seems like you took out most of the exercises from the Vol-1 DVD, so does that mean you are suppose to add the two volumes together?

- If we are only going to do the Vol-2 exercises now, that's a lot fewer exercises, since you are only doing the standing, lying down, BWEs, and the circles. Is that really all you need is just these, as it seems like doing more would do more? Are doing fewer exercises really building us up faster?

- On the new Vol-2 DVD you show us how to do the standing med with the new way of deep breathing, but I'm not sure which to breathe from, my nose or my mouth? Does it matter which way it is done, he looks like he does it with his nose, is that way better?

- Are you saying that doing this side-to-side, merry go round way of moving around the chi and not the top to bottom method is making it a spiritual exercise? I'm confused on how that makes it a spiritual exercise?

- Will either the Vol-1 or Vol-2 lead to us being able to levitate? Does your Inner Circle teach this technique? I really want to be able to do this, is it really possible?

- I'm starting to get a few rashes and reddish bumps on my bottom, knee caps and elbows, is this related to this training? Should I be concerned as it doesn't hurt or anything, it's just not attractive?

- Is there a difference between chi and the kundalini?

- One day I was moving my chi wheel w/my eyes by staring at the image thru the mirror, instead of the usual looking at it directly, how was that possible that I could still get it to move?

- Recently, I was moving around my chi spinner, trying to move it with as much power as I could and as fast as I could and suddenly a drawer opened up next to me w/o me touching it. Is it possible I could have done that or was it something else?

- My body usually gets very cold during and after the chi exercises and lasts for quite awhile after my workout. Is this a safe way to do these exercises? Is it okay to do the exercises in the cold the whole time or would it lead to bad side effects?

- On the Vol-2 Circle exercise, are you making the circles go around your entire body or just in front of the body? I can do it better if I'm the middle of the circle, is that okay? Is he showing the circles in front of him, at least that's what his arms are doing?

- I'm still a little skeptical yet, though I really am feeling a pickup of energy and these feeling of an electrical sensation, so I can see there is something to it. My question is how are you really gong to get us in touch with our spirits? I've been learning things from everywhere I can and nothing has worked yet, what are you doing that is different then the rest?

- I know it can vary as far as time, but I would like to know how long the normal person takes in order to feel their spirit for the first time?

- Sometimes, when I'm doing the fast blood washing exercise, after I'm finished and sitting there relaxing, I can feel this swirling sensation coming from different areas of my body. The funny thing is sometimes they go in the way you are teaching us, but sometimes they go the other way (counterclockwise) is this normal or am I doing the exercises wrong?

Q & A Session 8

- From listening to the Danger Zone MP3, I found out I was yanging, so I'm taking off a couple days like you suggested. My question is would it still be okay to listen to the MP3s on the Inner Circle website?

- Before I understood how bad it was to talk down to myself, I did it all the time. But now that I know better from the chi training you teach, I was wondering how I could see myself in a better way, so I don't do it so much. Any suggestions?

- I enjoyed the MP3 on Natural Killer Cells, so does this mean we should continue on with the energy packing & organ balancing exercises, as I want to keep my NK cells in great shape?

- I was wanting to get good at moving things like Sifu Andrei does and I was wondering if I put in an hour a day at trying to move something would I be able to do it quicker?

- I think I might have overloaded my organs, as I feel a slight pain pulsing from my kidneys and my spleen. It doesn't really hurt much, so I was wondering if I can still train? The pain isn't extreme like you're talking about.

- I'm coming in from a traditional yang style of chi gung and we did a lot of tightening exercises. The last few MP3s have made me re-think my views and I want to get on this yin side you're talking about. My question is how do I stop tightening up all the time as it just seems so natural to do it now?

- Concerning the pheromone MP3, I was wondering if someone is mad at you and triggers your hormones to get aggressive, how do you stop it from happening? I would think this is important, since your natural killer cells would be affected?

- I've heard from a bunch of sources now about the importance of protein, I thought they built muscles, is this something we should include in our diet? Does it matter which kind it is, either soy or whey, which is better?

- So, are you saying all we have to do is tell someone to turn their NK cells on in order for you to turn them on? Is it really that easy, as this doesn't seem like it could work?

- Does the moderate use of alcohol or any other type drugs inhibit significantly your chi training?

- Are you using the term nerve fibers to mean the same thing as the meridians that the Chinese refer to when speaking of the chi pathways?

- I really like the circle exercise and was wondering if we could do it longer than you show on Vol-2? Also is it alright to do the circles in the lying down meditation as I find I can do it very easily while doing it in that position? Is this a good way of doing the affirmations at night?

- A couple days ago, I was sitting up and relaxing, when I started to feel like I was vibrating (like a sphere), I went with the feeling for awhile, then when I opened my eyes the whole room was also vibrating like it had a breath or heartbeat to it. It lasted for several minutes. What's going on with that?

- Are you guys going to teach sparring with other chi persons using only pressure points and chi power without physically touching them?

- I know of a woman, who has severe health problems, issues with her heart and the only way she survives is by vampiring off other people's energies. Is this affecting those people like in the same way, when we get vampired on by those things that go bump in the night? What kind of energy does she absorb in order not to have a heart transplant?

Q & A Session 9

- Since you say it takes years, even for you guys, 2-3 yrs to get in touch with our spirit, will we be able to reach that point if we don't continue in the system past the first year? Do we have to be in the closed system part to learn this process?

- Is getting into the closed part of the system going to be an automatic process? Will there be other requirements?

- On using the chi stick, how do you know which way is up?

- Do you have any other tips on how to handle the sexual energy build up, as it seems to build in me to unreal levels no matter which way I do it, any suggestions?

- I work on new people everyday (from 1-3 daily) and I was wondering what I should do when one of those people walk in all yanged out, as it has a tendency right now to be very draining and adversely affecting me?

- Could you explain in a little more detail how you put the good feeling energy into the blob of energy we move around? I feel the blob of energy, but don't get how to make it (the blob itself) feel good?

- Can you explain about the seven vortexes a little more, as I think I activated one in my chi point area? That whole area will just spontaneously start spinning sometime during my workout, making me feel the weirdest sensations, is this suppose to feel this way? Sometimes I feel it, and I'm not even working out.

- I was wondering what is happening with me lately, It started out by me feeling these waves of energy coming thru my body as I listened to the 8th month video on affirmations, but now when I listen to any of the mp3s (even by other certified instructors) this wave feeling continues to happen. Is that a normal thing?

- If I wanted to manifest something with a training partner would it still work okay, even though he's moving away to a different state? Does the distance matter?

- Do we as Inner Circle Members, need to purchase a Chi Stick? It's kind of expensive, so if we don't need it, I just soon not have to buy it.

- I have a question concerning magnets. Does the use of magnets benefit your training that much? I'm curious, as I see them advertised a lot of places and notice you occasionally sell them. If they are worth the money I'll get them, but would like your opinion first.

- You have mentioned the term inflows and outflows a couple times now, but I still don't know what this means. Are you talking about using the breaths or is this that body breathing you're talking about?

- I have studied about how to do a Dim Mak technique for 10-yrs now and was wondering if I got your Dim Mak course, if it would give me the missing pieces of the puzzle I seem to be missing? Will your course really teach me to do a death touch?

- Can you explain to me how to give someone an autosuggestion that would work, even though they may be across the country away?

Interviews with Certified Instructors

The "Interviews with the Certified Instructors" are some of the most valuable nuggets of information within the Inner Circle. Here you will find very candid discussions between Master Instructors Sifu Jones and Sifu Perhacs, and the Certified Instructors they have trained over the years. The conversations are real; the atmosphere is open and; although somewhat fantastic, the statements made regarding each of their personal journeys and experiences with the chi are the acme of truth.

Members of the Inner Circle have the opportunity to listen to these Interviews at their leisure, as often as they like, and even ask questions to the Master Instructors for additional insight so as to maximize their personal training. The opportunities to avoid pitfalls and accentuate that which is euphoric are the takeaways of each Interview; and each Instructor brings a perspective and experience that is diverse as the Inner Circle itself. There is something (lots of things) for everyone.

Sifu Michael Allen

Sifu Michael Allen began training with Sifu Jones in 1995. His martial arts background was mixed: traditional karate; ju jutsu; judo; hapkido; and Chinese boxing with Sifu Jones.

Like most of us, Michael Allen looked for chi training his entire life, and as he tells the Inner Circle of the few instances he found people who could demonstrate various levels of psi related abilities, none offered an approach like that found within Chi Power, as taught by Sifu Jones.

Michael's background was atypically "yang". He admits he and his entire family were all "tough guys", and fisticuffs were the norm. A natural to chi, he tells the Inner Circle of how is own ion shield protected him from a conflagration when a wood-burning stove erupted inches from his face. In fact, many of Michael Allen's experiences are hard to comprehend, but as many of us know from firsthand experience, fact is far more fantastic than fiction.

Michael warns the Inner Circle of the hazards that come with over training. In fact, he is one of the few Chi Power practitioners to get negative side effects (read painful energy spikes resulting in organ pain) from doing the yin exercises too long; he would spend anywhere between 18 to 36 hours mastering deep meditation techniques that would lead to bizarre Out of Body Experiences you have to listen for yourself to fully grasp. In his own words, they were often "very disconcerting".

He warns the members of the Inner Circle to follow the curriculum, and most importantly, trust and listen to the instructions set forth by Sifu Jones and Sifu Perhacs, as the goal is to assist our chi progression without having to go thru the physical pain he (Michael Allen) experienced.

Sifu Benjamin Richardson

Benjamin Richardson began his training with Sifu Jones in 1997. He is one of the "original mavericks", taking the concept of "yang" to new levels.

Sifu Richardson's background is wrought with chi gung exploration. Having studied *Wing Chun* in his youth, he used his time in the Navy to travel the world looking for masters to teach him the secrets of chi.

Sifu Richardson details his experiences, the good and the bad, to assist the members of the Inner Circle along their individual path. He conveys his personal challenges and the telltale signs of "yanging" are conveyed with a stunning contrast of how wonderful his life has become since he embraced Sifu Jones' concept of being *yin*.

Sifu Richardson shares with us the various esoteric styles of breathing techniques and some of the more unusual training practices he encountered. Members of the Inner Circle who listen to Sifu Richardson's even, cool, very calm and euphoric tones will know that he is providing a roadmap to help those new to this method avoid unnecessary pitfalls and very, very real pains.

Sifu Andrei Biesinger

Andrei Biesinger has been training with Sifu Jones and Sifu Perhacs in the year 2004. His background is that of a natural healer, and has a mind that is without bounds. Andrei's energy and enthusiasm is the kind that "gets the party started". He does not mince words, nor does he hold back. His experiences are truly amazing: from healing his own broken ankle and walking on it later the same night to using his chi to find his ideal house, Andrei takes the lofty, enigmatic concepts of chi and applies them in very concrete ways which he demonstrates personally.

Featured in several videos, Andrei demonstrates his uncanny sensitivity and chi manipulation in ways that boggle the mind. From bending spoons to sensing [different] objects to sharing with us his experiences with chi, Andrei gives members of the Inner Circle a glimpse into the possibilities of their own future.

Sifu Charles Dragoo

Sifu Charles Dragoo began training with Sifu Jones in 1989. Like many others, he was a "yang" maverick, and actually blended the SPC USA Chi Power Method with the practices of other chi gung practitioners. Members of the Inner Circle will find his extremely painful experiences of great interest and significant importance, knowing the results of said practices and avoiding it completely.

Sifu Dragoo has had the distinct opportunity to train with some very well known chi gung practitioners over his lifetime, and shares with us his experiences with Jane Hallander and others.

Charles also details the limitations and painful (and sometimes odd) side effects of the "Lin Kung Jing" (empty force). From setting off alarms in stores; causing windows to slam shut as he walked past; to accidentally hurting his own [Wing Chun] students, Sifu Charles Dragoo has truly experienced the yang "roller coaster" ride and is more than pleased now that he has found the euphoria of *yin* training.

Sifu Don Brown

Don Brown began his training with Sifu Jones and Sifu Perhacs in 1998. His background is an amalgam of intellectual curiosity, stemming from his introduction to the concept of chi in martial arts [tai chi] and similarities between the two.

Don is featured on a number of Interviews with Master Instructors, Sifu Jones and Sifu Perhacs regarding scientific discoveries and chi. Don's scientific curiosity, background in Engineering (Masters of Science in Information Sciences) and [admitted] skeptical nature make him a perfect research assistant for the Inner Circle.

Don's interviews focus on the following subjects and how the latest scientific data correlate to chi, and more specifically, Chi Power: quantum physics; pheromones; natural killer cells; chi and the brain; emotional content and hormone. The information conveyed therein is backed with hours upon hours of research, and is explained in layman terms; Don and Sifu Jones take great strides in not "dumbing it down", but more importantly, step by step, educating you on the nuances of each topic, so that a complete and thorough understanding of the information can be shared by the Inner Circle, and incorporated into our daily lives.

Chapter 6: The Closed Door

In his book <u>Entangled Minds,</u> Dean Radin provides a very accurate view into the nature and necessity of the secrecy involved within the Closed Door System. It is a *welcome* that contains within a caution:

> "In a society that seeks out and cultivates people with natural psi talent, and cares for their special sensitivities, it's conceivable that groups with refined psi abilities could prosper. Such groups might prove to be extremely useful to society. Unfortunately, it's also likely that the existence of such groups would introduce intense fear and resentment in those who were less gifted, and it isn't clear that such a group could be controlled for very long by *outsiders*. Thus, if such a group *were* formed, they'd have to be established under conditions of extreme secrecy."

Behind the Closed Door

Members of the Inner Circle who take the lessons and instruction provided by Master Instructors Sifu Jones and Sifu Perhacs can look forward to an invitation to the Closed Door System.

Whereas the Chi Power System is akin to traditional chi gung on steroids, the exercises and techniques taught in the Closed Door System are exponentially more intense. The margin for error decreases significantly as the throughput of the energy increases at an alarming rate.

Although inklings of the power within began to manifest during the 1st year of the Inner Circle, here behind the Closed Door, select students will have the opportunity to master these abilities and techniques, and perform not only at a higher level at all times, but more importantly: with control, and on demand.

Two 6 Month Intensive Training Systems

The Closed Door System is comprised of a two 6-month intensive training system, comprised of (1) one module per month. Accompanying each module is an online forum, moderated by Certified Instructors as well as Master Instructors Sifu Jones and Sifu Perhacs, where students can discuss side effects, experiences and ask questions not only of the Sifus, but of each other.

Within these modules are the specific techniques that teach the extreme abilities that draw upon many of our fancies: levitation; moving objects without touching them; out of body experiences and astral projection, to name a few.

The 1st 6 Months (Form Chi)

The 1st 6 Month System of the Closed Door System, introduces the Chi Power practitioner to static/formed chi via the Volume 3 Advanced DVD: How to Form Static Chi.

These exercises cause an exponential increase in the *density* of the chi, making it so physically tangible that it can be formed into specific shapes by the mind and hold said shapes for use in very advanced techniques.

Please note: during this phase of training, the importance of keeping the energy cool and euphoric cannot be stressed enough; it is during this phase of the training that many of the Certified Instructors encountered amplified organ pain and terrors of "yanging out".

Closed Door: Module One (Release of Advanced Chi DVD Volume 3)

The first module opens with the **Volume 3 Advanced DVD**. Accompanying the Volume 3 DVD is a manual which provides additional training instructions and information on how the process of forming static chi is achieved.

Also provided is a detailed .mp3 that walks the trainee thru the process, step-by-step, ensuring proper form and desired results.

A [web-based] forum will be available for the Closed System members, giving them an opportunity to discuss their training amongst their peers. This forum also serves as a vehicle for the Sifus to provide additional information between monthly topics.

Closed Door: ModuleTwo (Body Breathing)

During the second module, **"Body Breathing Part-2"** is introduced. The body breathing method is explained in detail, how this process will occur. This one method is so secretive and is rarely taught to outsiders in most Closed Systems.

Closed Door: Module Three (Advanced OBE)

During the third module, **Advanced Training on OBEs** begins. This process will allow the practitioner to learn how to control the OBE process. In the past the OBE's are more a "pop out" sequence with less control. In this training, you will begin to merge even more of the Mind, Body and Spirit.

Closed Door: Module Four (Wall to Wall Exercise)

During the fourth module, students are taught the "**Wall to Wall Exercise**", where they learn to use their chi forms in very specific and advanced ways.

Closed Door: Module Five (Advanced Circle Training)

The fifth module introduces **Advanced Circle Exercises**, where the student learns how incorporate forms in conjunction to their circles. Although this is generally done with a chi-stick, instruction will be provided for those without chi-sticks to help them get the same results as those who use the chi-stick.

Closed Door: Module Six (Levitation 101)

The sixth month offers the instruction for which many have been waiting: Levitation 101. This is also the student's introduction to the upper echelon of the Water Stage, where the beginning aspects of fasting are taught as it directly impacts this level training.

The 2nd 6 Months Closed Door System (Super Set Training)

The 2nd 6 Months of the Closed Door System introduces *"super sets"* via the **Advanced Chi Power DVD Volume 4 Vol-4: The Super Sets.** This set of exercises guide the practitioner thru the next part of learning to form chi and create enough speed to create vortexes.

Like the First 6 months, there will also be a forum where students can interact with one another via the web, to share experiences and the like.

These forums are deliberately separate from one another; it is important that only those who are mentally, physically, and emotionally ready for the second module of the Closed Door System to share and interact at that level. Exposure to this training and information too soon adversely affects the adept's progress.

Closed Door: Module Seven (Effective Control Methods)

During the seventh module, an .mp3 on **"How to get an effective control over these new exercises and what to expect next from the training"** becomes available. The instructions therein provide guidance concerning the best ways to do the *super sets* for maximum results.

Closed Door: Module Eight (Liquid Chi)

Module Eight introduces the concept of and provides instructions on how to create *liquid chi.*

An .mp3 on how this new set of exercises changes the way chi interacts with the fabric of reality, as well as the time-space distortions (and other pleasantly strange side effects) our Certified Instructions candidly shared during Inner Circle interviews.

Closed Door: Module Nine (Hypnotic Devices Training)

The Ninth Module begins the incorporation of hypnotic devices which, in turn, amplify the chi via engaging the student's mind that much deeper.

With an even greater, deliberate focus, members of the Closed Door System learn to build chi at an alarming rate: just five minutes a time. Welcome to "Poster Training".

Closed Door: Module Ten (Super Set Variations)

The tenth module introduces variations of the Super Sets and provides the cues as when to change the exercises in order to keep moving forward; this enables members of the Closed Door System to bypass the plateau that so many others reach early in their chi training.

Closed Door: Module Eleven (Fractal Images)

During Module Eleven of the Closed Door System, Fractal Images are introduced. Beyond the geometric mathematical concepts, their significance to chi and how they are used is explained in great detail.

Many of the extreme psi-related abilities are a result of properly using fractal images in conjunction with formed chi and vortexes.

Closed Door: Module Twelve (Integration of All Techiques)

The Twelveth Module of the Closed Door System provides a means for students to receive their Black Belt in our Circular Yin Style. The requirements are made known via an .mp3 and video.

Please understand: although the curriculum of the Closed Door System is safe, the practice of the techniques therein is very similar to the nature of the traditional martial arts dojo.

Within traditional martial arts, from karate to kung fu, the student actively participates in an atmosphere of *controlled violence*. An alert and focused mind on the part of everyone within the dojo is that which allows the student to safely walk that fine line of "training" as opposed to sustaining life-debilitating injuries.

So is it with the Closed Door System. Increased monitoring of the students' psychological and physical well-being requires greater interaction with the Certified Instructors as well as greater vigilance from the Master Instructors and, most importantly: a commitment to excellence from each and every student!

Scientific Premium Company-USA Products

All of our products are of the highest quality and contain methods not found elsewhere…These courses will provide a foundation to getting into the CHI POWER INNER CIRCLE.

Chi Power Plus

Our original course in either electronic or hard copy form.
http://masterthepower.com/chi_power_plus.html

Advanced Chi Training System

This contains all of our courses at an incredible value. Our top selling products.
http://masterthepower.com/act_upgrade.htm
To receive all updates and stay current with what is going on with Chi Power Training, please visit our **Chi Power Syndicate Blog**, which is updated regularly.
http://www.chipower.com/blog

Mind Force Collection of Esoteric Products

http://www.mindforcesecrets.com
Guided Meditation, Remote Viewing, Astral Projection, OBE (Mind Portal)
http://mindforcesecrets.com/mind_portal.php

Psychic Energy Development & Power (Internal Power Centers)
http://mindforcesecrets.com/ipc.php

Law of Attraction & Manifestation (The Magneto Method)
http://mindforcesecrets.com/magneto.php

Hypnosis, Self Hypnosis, Covert Persuasion (Closed Door Hypnosis Files)
http://mindforcesecrets.com/closed_door.php

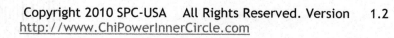

CPSIA information can be obtained
at www.ICGtesting.com
Printed in the USA
LVOW03s1920211216
518291LV00022B/326/P